Clinical Research: From Proposal to Implementation

Clinical Research: From Proposal to Implemention

Michael J. McPhaul, MD
Department of Internal Medicine
Division of Endocrinology
The University of Texas Southwestern Medical Center at Dallas
Dallas, Texas

Robert D. Toto, MD
Department of Internal Medicine
Division of Nephrology
The University of Texas Southwestern Medical Center at Dallas
Dallas, Texas

Research Ethics Commentaries by
Simon J. Craddock Lee, PhD, MPH and John Z. Sadler, MD

Wolters Kluwer | Lippincott Williams & Wilkins
Health
Philadelphia · Baltimore · New York · London
Buenos Aires · Hong Kong · Sydney · Tokyo

Acquisitions Editor: Sonya Seigafuse
Product Manager: Kerry Barrett
Production Manager: Alicia Jackson
Senior Manufacturing Manager: Benjamin Rivera
Marketing Manager: Kim Schonberger
Design Coordinator: Holly McLaughlin
Production Service: MPS Limited, A Macmillan Company

Library of Congress Cataloging-in-Publication Data

Clinical research : from proposal to implementation / edited by Michael J. McPhaul, Robert D. Toto; ethical commentaries by Simon J. Craddock Lee and John Z. Sadler.
   p. ; cm.
   Includes bibliographical references and index.
   Summary: "Clinical and translational research is a crucial link to the improvement of clinical care and practice. Many of the elements that are involved—physicians, nurses, pharmacists, laboratory testing, medical records—are also involved in the delivery of care to patients. Yet in the conduct of clinical research, these elements are arrayed in different configurations and constrained by rules and regulations that are distinct from those that guide the practice of medicine. In parallel with these considerations, the conduct of clinical research demands a specific skill set. Specialized tools are required to formulate and design informative clinical trials and to interpret the findings from such experiments"—Provided by publisher.
   ISBN-13: 978-1-60547-748-0 (alk. paper)
   ISBN-10: 1-60547-748-6 (alk. paper)
   1. Clinical trials. I. McPhaul, Michael J. II. Toto, Robert D.
   [DNLM: 1. Biomedical Research—methods. 2. Clinical Trials as Topic—methods. 3. Research Design.
   W 20.5 C64115 2011]
   R853.C55C55 2011
   615.5072'4—dc22

                             2010021684

To purchase additional copies of this book, call our customer service department at (800) 638-3030 or fax orders to (301) 223-2320. International customers should call (301) 223-2300.

Visit Lippincott Williams & Wilkins on the Internet: at LWW.com. Lippincott Williams & Wilkins customer service representatives are available from 8:30 am to 6 pm, EST.

10 9 8 7 6 5 4 3 2 1

CCS0810

To Amanda and to my family, for their support and love.
To my father, John, and my mother, Marilyn.
MJM

To my dear and loving wife for her thoughtfulness
and unswerving support throughout my career.
RDT

Clinical and translational research is a crucial link to the improvement of clinical care and practice. Many of the elements that are involved—physicians, nurses, pharmacists, laboratory testing, medical records—are also involved in the delivery of care to patients. Yet in the conduct of clinical research, these elements are arrayed in different configurations and constrained by rules and regulations that are distinct from those that guide the practice of medicine. In parallel with these considerations, the conduct of clinical research demands a specific skill set. Specialized tools are required to formulate and design informative clinical trials and to interpret the findings from such experiments.

To address these needs, institutions have established didactic programs to train research personnel in disciplines ranging from experimental design, to statistics, to the ethics of research. Despite the availability of these important resources at many institutions, such training is not uniformly available. Further, even within institutions at which such training is readily available, we have perceived a need for a basic guide designed to facilitate the recognition of basic potential roadblocks and to help identify the critical elements and resources necessary to transform a research proposal into an active research protocol. During the evolution of our own clinical research training programs, we identified a gap between completing the writing of a clinical research protocol and implementing the protocol in the research environment. This book is an attempt to fill that gap. We anticipate that teachers, students, and experienced investigators will find this book extremely valuable in understanding and improving the conduct and completion of clinical and translational research studies.

CONTENTS

Robert D. Toto, MD

Suzanne M. Rivera, PhD

Anne Clark, CIP, Suzanne M. Rivera, PhD, MSW, P. Diane Sheppard, RN, Darren K. McGuire, MD, MHSc, and Michael J. McPhaul, MD

CHAPTER 4   Ethics of Data Sharing and Handling of Genetic Information   41

Bradley A. Malin, PhD, David Karp, MD, PhD, and Richard H. Scheuermann, PhD

CHAPTER 5   Writing a Statistical Analysis Plan   57

Beverley Adams-Huet, MS and Chul Ahn, PhD

CHAPTER 6   Protocol Implementation Procedures   72

Tammy L. Lightfoot, RN, BSN

CHAPTER 7   Screening and Evaluation   77

CHAPTER 8   Recruitment and Retention   86

CHAPTER 9   How to Set up Your Database   97

CHAPTER 10   Budgeting Process and Management   113

CHAPTER 11   Understanding Food and Drug Administration (FDA) Regulatory Requirements for Investigational New Drug Applications (IND) for Sponsor-Investigators   132

M. E. Blair Holbein, PhD

CHAPTER 12   Collecting Data   147

Deanna S. Adams, RN

CHAPTER 13   Data and Safety Monitoring   163

Andrea M. Nassen, RN, MSN

CONTRIBUTING AUTHORS

Deanna S. Adams, RN
Regulatory Specialist
Department of Clinical Sciences
UT Southwestern Medical Center at Dallas
Dallas, Texas

Beverley Adams-Huet, MS
Assistant Professor
Department of Clinical Sciences, Division
    of Biostatistics
University of Texas Southwestern Medical
    Center
Dallas, Texas

Chul Ahn, PhD
Professor, Director of Biostatistics and
    Research Design
Department of Clinical Sciences
University of Texas Southwestern Medical
    Center
Dallas, Texas

Anne Clark, CIP
Senior IRB Coordinator
Institutional Review Board/Research Services
UT Southwestern
Dallas, Texas

Simon J. Craddock Lee, PhD, MPH
Assistant Professor of Clinical Sciences
    (Medical Anthropology)
Department of Clinical Sciences
Division of Ethics & Health Policy
University of Texas Southwestern Medical
    Center
Member
Population Science and Cancer Control
Harold C. Simmons Cancer Center
Dallas, Texas

M. E. Blair Holbein, PhD
Assistant Professor
Department of Clinical Sciences
Director, Clinical Investigator Resource Core
University of Texas Southwestern Medical
    Center
Dallas, Texas

David R. Karp, MD, PhD
Professor
Department of Internal Medicine
University of Texas Southwestern Medical
    Center
Dallas, Texas

Tammy L. Lightfoot, RN, BSN
Clinical Research Manager
Department of Internal Medicine, Division
    of Nephrology
University of Texas Southwestern Medical
    Center at Dallas
Dallas, Texas

Bradley A. Malin, PhD
Assistant Professor
Department of Biomedical Informatics
Vanderbilt University
Nashville, Tennessee

Darren K. McGuire, MD, MHSc
Associate Professor
Department of Internal Medicine-Cardiology
University of Texas Southwestern Medical
    Center at Dallas
Medical Director
Cardiology Clinics
Parkland Hospital and Health System
Dallas, Texas

Michael J. McPhaul, MD
Professor
Department of Internal Medicine, Division
    of Endocrinology
University of Texas Southwestern Medical
    Center
Dallas, Texas

Andrea M. Nassen, RN, MSN
Research Participant Advocate
Department of Clinical Sciences
UT Southwestern Medical Center
Dallas, Texas

Suzanne M. Rivera, PhD, MSW
Assistant Professor
Department of Clinical Sciences
UT Southwestern Medical School
Vice President
Research Administration
UT Southwestern Medical Center
Dallas, Texas

A. John Rush, MD
Professor and Vice Dean
Clinical Sciences
Duke-NUS Graduate Medical School
Singapore

John Z. Sadler, MD
Professor of Psychiatry and Clinical Sciences
Chief
Division of Ethics & Health Policy
Department of Clinical Sciences
The University of Texas Southwestern
    Medical Center
Dallas, Texas

Richard H. Scheuermann, PhD
Professor
Department of Pathology
Chief, Division of Biomedical Informatics
Department of Clinical Sciences
U.T. Southwestern Medical Center
Dallas, Texas

P. Diane Sheppard, RN
Manager, Institutional Review Board
Research Services
University of Texas Southwestern at Dallas,
Dallas Texas

Janet P. Smith, BA
Manager, Database Applications
    Development
Clinical Sciences, Division of Biostatistics
UT Southwestern Medical Center
Dallas, Texas

Charles T. Quinn, MD, MS
Associate Professor of Clinical Pediatrics
Department of Pediatrics
University of Cincinnati College of
    Medicine
Director of Hematology Clinical and
    Translational Research
Department of Hematology -Oncology
Cincinnati Children's Hospital Medical
    Center
Cincinnati, Ohio

Robert D. Toto, MD
Department of Internal Medicine
Division of Nephrology
The University of Texas Southwestern
    Medical Center at Dallas
Dallas, Texas

How to Launch a Successful Career in Clinical Research: Tips on Making the Most of Available Resources

Robert D. Toto, MD

INTRODUCTION

An important part of implementing any clinical research study is to have the time, resources, and mind-set to publish the final results of the study. This review is focused on some practical aspects of how young investigators may avail themselves of the resources needed to launch and sustain a successful career in clinical research. The three elements focused on here are finding protected time, the importance of mentorship, and practical tips for publishing results.

FINDING AND PROTECTING TIME TO CONDUCT CLINICAL RESEARCH

One of the most precious commodities for a clinical researcher is creation of protected time for research **(Table 1-1)**. Achieving and maintaining ample time to conduct a clinical research project and publish it requires thoughtful input by the researcher and his or her mentor(s). Many young clinical investigators are talented individuals who have little training in research methods and may have competing responsibilities that can hinder the implementation and

1

T A B L E   **1-1** | **Tips for Finding Protected Time to Conduct Clinical Research**

- Meet with your chief, and discuss your career plans
- Decide how you want to spend your time for the next 5 years
- Obtain commitment to pursue research and develop a realistic plan
- Avail yourself of relevant resources (e.g., General Clinical Research Center)
- Focus your "free" time on research project(s)
- Minimize clinical service time (25% or less)
- Minimize administrative work
- Limit lectures to those that serve to foster your research career
- Presentation or attendance at local, regional, and national meetings that advertise your work
- Avoid writing manuscripts unrelated to your research

completion of a research project. For example, clinical responsibilities for patient care or teaching junior trainees in a medical or graduate school take time that might otherwise be spent conducting research. Many young investigators are comfortable with teaching or, in the case of physicians, with direct patient care or patient administrative activities as part of their previous training but are not so comfortable with research activities. Young and energetic researchers are assets to their departments and often receive requests to spend time on non-research activities that they are often quite comfortable with. For example, junior faculty and postdoctoral fellows training in or beginning a career in clinical research may be tempted to use their talents to help others and will be highly sought after by superiors, colleagues, and others to do administrative work, run and/or attend to clinics, see more patients, provide coverage, and serve on committees. To the greatest extent possible, these activities should be minimized to maximize time for research. The decision to accept new or additional clinical and administrative responsibilities is an important one for those beginning a career in clinical research and should be discussed with their mentor and department chairperson or division chief. In general, when it is an "optional" (e.g., request from colleague) activity, then the decision should be based on whether it will benefit one's research plan and career. For example, preparing a lecture on a topic directly related to one's own research question or project might be time well spent in that it can have a direct and positive impact on a future publication in one's own field of research.

An important step before implementing a research project is to exact the protected time that is needed to successfully carry out the project including the writing and publishing of the final manuscript. To accomplish this, it is ideal for a young researcher to meet with their department chairperson or division chief, preferably with their mentor present to discuss their career plans and have a clear outline of expectations on how one's time will be spent over the next 5 years. Obtaining a commitment for protected time to conduct research from one's department chairperson should be done up front before project development to maximize the likelihood of one's success as a researcher and ultimately for academic advancement. This discussion should include some details of what the research project will entail and if the plans of the researcher and their mentor are congruent with the goals of the department. This is extremely valuable not only for the researcher but also for the department or division head.

Learn to Say No!

It is important for individuals to learn to say no to requests for non–research-related activities when the time commitment is substantial, and the benefit is questionable or not palpable, for example, preparing a lecture that is unrelated to the research project at hand. Delivering a lecture may take less than an hour, but preparation time may take 20 to 40 hours depending on the topic when considering researching the topic, writing and practicing the lecture, and, finally, making the presentation. In addition, to learning to say no when asked to perform less productive activities, those apart from research, a researcher should avail themselves of all available resources. These can include local, regional, and national resources that apply to the research question and research project including local environmental resources such as a National Institutes of Health–funded clinical research center. A few hints on how to maintain protected time include (1) focusing "free" time on research project(s); (2) minimizing clinical service time (for physicians, no more than 25%); (3) minimizing administrative duties (e.g., declining invitations to serve on non–research-related committees); and (4) limiting lectures to those that foster one's research career. In addition, opportunities to write book chapters, editorials, and review articles that deviate from one's main research topic should, in most cases, be avoided. In contrast, preparing and delivering presentations to patients and health care providers that may foster recruitment and or retain study participants is time well spent. Similarly, presentations or attendance at regional and national meetings that serve to promote research represent activities in which one's participation makes good use of time. Finally, an article that is a critical review of literature central to one's research hypothesis or a paper on the study design of an ongoing research project is an example of time well spent by a young investigator.

A Positive Approach

A positive approach to clinical research training is to look at it as a challenge and an opportunity. Those who choose to pursue research as a career have already achieved much success as undergraduates, graduates, and house staff (MDs). Still, the challenges of training and pursuing a research career can be daunting and may necessitate overcoming anxiety and insecurity, or fear of failure. A suggested approach is to take the view that research training is a process that provides new and exciting opportunities for professional and personal growth. Preventing or overcoming anxiety related to the prospect of succeeding in a research project can be achieved by keeping a positive outlook, not worrying about what might be and having faith in one's abilities and the environment. In addition, the thought of finishing a project and seeing it published inspires and creates a sense of satisfaction, self-worth, and, for some, relief.

WORK CLOSELY WITH MENTORS

Identifying and working closely with a mentor can be both rewarding and productive not only for junior but also for senior investigators. Many investigators develop and maintain healthy relationships with mentors throughout their careers, although one may have more than one mentor at any given time, and the mentor(s) may change over time. A mentor

RESEARCH ETHICS: PITFALLS & PRESCRIPTIONS

As essential as mentor–mentee relationships are, they often pose troubling ethical questions for early investigators. Because the mentee is "one-down" in power, disagreements—scientific or ethical—are difficult for mentees to raise and discuss. Mentors, on the other hand, may find themselves in awkward situations when a mentee is failing to produce, or neglecting work. Frank discussion at the beginning of the relationship can address how to handle disagreement, and how to address lack of progress should it occur.

Detsky AS, Baerlocher, MO. Academic mentoring—how to give it and how to get it. *JAMA.* 2007;297:2134–2136.

provides many tangibles and intangibles of value to those planning a career in research. For example, some mentors are inspirational and charismatic. Charismatic or not, they stimulate young investigators to pursue research in areas that they are passionate about. Mentors also provide important intellectual input and critique of one's approach or interpretation of research data. They challenge mentees to ask important questions and develop methods to answer such questions that can help to build a research career. Mentors serve as advocates for mentees in a variety of ways including eking out and maintaining protected time for research endeavors; introducing mentees to other leaders in the field; and helping them to obtain recognition for their work at local, regional, national, and international levels. Mentors also assist mentees in academic advancement within their institution, in grant applications for research funding and research publications, and in finding full-time jobs. Characteristics of a good mentor include the ability to teach—a person within an institution that is respected and trusted by his/her peers in the research community and one who himself/herself is an accomplished researcher. Finally, a key feature of a good mentor is one who is accessible. A mentee will have little success with a mentor if the mentor is relatively inaccessible. Accessing a mentor as often as needed is ideal, but in general, early on in training, a mentee should access his or her mentor at least once a week to review data, progress on a project, monitor career development, and solve problems.

Roles of the Mentor and the Mentee

The mentor–mentee relationship is first and foremost a professional relationship that is a two-way street **(Table 1-2)**. Both parties benefit from a working relationship in similar ways. For example, both may benefit by working together on a research project that culminates in a publication that changes clinical practice. The mentor must also be a promoter, a protector, as well as a challenger and empathizer, and advocate for the mentee in many spheres including those mentioned above (e.g., protected time and academic advancement). The mentee's roles and responsibilities include having self-awareness about what they desire in the future and what drives them. Understanding these is very important in the mentor–mentee relationship and should be openly discussed with the mentor at the earliest point in the relationship. This self-awareness helps both parties understand how to best

TABLE **1-2** | **Mentor and Mentee Relationships**

Role and Responsibilities of Mentor	Role and Responsibilities of Mentee
• Inspiration	• Self-awareness
• Intellectual input/critique/challenge	• Be open with mentor about career plans, needs, wants, etc.
• Protection of time for research	• Prepare before meeting with mentor
• Recognition—local, regional, national, and international	• Set expectations and review progress regularly
• Academic advancement	• Be fierce about your work, work hard, and persevere
• Funding	• Exercise discipline and perseverance
• Success in publication	• Stay focused on research question
• Success in promotion and finding position	• Know strengths and limitations

plan the career development of the mentee. Therefore, having an open relationship with the mentor concerning career plans, needs, and wants is an important responsibility of the mentee. A mentee should therefore be prepared and set expectations before his/her meeting with a mentor and thereafter set expectations and review progress regularly (e.g., weekly). Ultimately, success of the mentee requires both discipline and perseverance and being fierce about one's work. Meeting with one's mentor weekly to discuss ideas, protocol problems, data, and troubleshooting is very important for starting and staying focused on the protocol at hand. Productivity in these meetings can be enhanced by the mentee reading voraciously both in his/her own field (~90%) and in disparate fields (~10%). Conducting one's own research project under the tutelage of a strong mentor enhances the intellectual growth, acquisition of new skills, and elaboration of underlying talents while, at the same time, helping the mentee to understand his/her strengths and limitations. Valuable lessons can be learned from close professional relationships with one's mentors.

Learning from the Research Team

In addition to learning aspects of research design, new knowledge in the field, and practical information from one's mentor, members of a research team are a valuable resource for implementing a research protocol. For example, one may learn a great deal about patient recruitment and good clinical practice from a senior research nurse. This experience is extremely important for those who wish to conduct clinical trials. Collaborating researchers are another source of educational value for a young investigator conducting a new research protocol. Some collaborators may become comentors to mentees who wish to expand their expertise at some point in their career. Engaging clinicians who care for the study population of interest either through direct patient contact or through educational seminars is another way one can enhance recruitment and recruitment skills. In addition, whenever possible, optimally on a regular basis, one-on-one meetings with a biostatistician are another way a young investigator should avail himself/herself of an important learning process (see Chapter 5). Other members of a study team such as a database manager and a pharmacist can also teach mentees aspects of protocol implementation that a mentor may not be familiar or facile with. In summary, a young investigator should avail himself/herself of all human resources possible on the road to implementing a research proposal.

PUBLISHING YOUR RESULTS

The central and most important goal of a research project is to get the results published regardless of whether the findings are those predicted in the beginning and regardless of whether the results are "positive" or "negative." During the protocol implementation, it is desirable to begin to think about publishing the results and, in fact, envisioning how the final paper will actually appear in print **(Table 1-3)**. One can ask oneself "How will my final paper look when published?" It is helpful to revisit the research question posed and what the message of the paper will be in the end. Keeping this in mind helps one to conduct the research protocol properly that, in turn, helps to ensure the validity of the findings at study end.

It is not premature to think about publishing results before a study is completed. For some young investigators, writing clearly and scientifically is challenging and can sometimes lead to procrastination in getting studies published. One can begin the process of writing the final paper during the protocol implementation and completion. A first step in this process is to write an outline of the manuscript and then begin to fill in the spaces. One may not realize it, but a substantial portion of the manuscript is written in the protocol. For example, the methods section of the protocol can be used as a template for the methods section of the paper. In addition, the background and significance of the research protocol becomes a template for the introduction and may lend itself in part to the discussion section of the paper pending the results. Although the results section cannot be written, one can begin to create shells for tables and figures. For instance, a table of the participant characteristics in a clinical trial or observational study can be constructed in preparation for input of data later on. Also, one can catalog the key references that will be used in the introduction, methods, and discussion sections of the manuscript, and many, if not most, are in the references to the protocol or are part of the body of literature reviewed by the

T A B L E   **1-3** | Tips for Publishing Results: What You Can Do Ahead of Time

- Outline manuscript
- Use study protocol as template
- Create templates for tables and figures
- Use your protocol
- Think about presentation of results
- Create templates for tables and figures
- Collect and catalog key references along the way
- One manuscript—one message

investigator when preparing the protocol. Finally, one can consider several potential journals where the future manuscript may be submitted, and formatting for the selected journal can begin ahead of time. These are time-saving tips for getting ready to publish the manuscript later on when the data are collected, analyzed, and interpreted. These ideas are developed more completely in Chapter 14.

In summary, young investigators need research resources including protected time mentors and materials and a study team to successfully conduct a clinical research project. Finding the time for research, working closely with mentors, and thinking about publishing results early on are important aspects to future success in clinical research.

CHAPTER 2

Institutional Review Board Approval

Suzanne M. Rivera, PhD

OUTLINE

INTRODUCTION

The conduct of clinical trials is a complicated process that includes safeguards for study subjects and trial investigators. Researchers and study sponsors are required to comply with a myriad of regulations enforced by numerous oversight entities. The Federal Policy for the Protection of Human Subjects (45CFR§46) issued by the Department of Health and Human Services (DHHS) governs biomedical, social, and behavioral research. These regulations, first promulgated in 1981, have become the U.S. national standard for the conduct of human research. Having now been adopted by other federal agencies, the policy usually is referred to as *The Common Rule*. All institutions (domestic and international) that accept U.S. federal dollars for human research must assure, via a binding agreement with the DHHS, that they will comply with the Common Rule. This chapter focuses on the role of the Institutional Review Board (IRB) in the conduct of clinical trials.

WHAT IS AN IRB?

The Common Rule requires that research involving human subjects must be reviewed by a committee called an IRB. According to the federal definition, human research "means a systematic investigation, including research development, testing and evaluation, designed to develop or contribute to generalizable knowledge and which uses living humans or identifiable information about living humans" (1). This definition includes everything from randomized clinical trials to questionnaires. At universities and hospitals, virtually all research done with people, or with private information about people, is subject to IRB review.

Institutional review boards are committees that review and oversee human research studies. At universities and hospitals, IRBs are comprised mostly of physician researchers, nonphysician scientists, and administrative personnel, such as attorneys and risk managers. Frequently, allied health professionals, such as nurses and social workers, also participate. In addition, federal regulations require that each IRB must have at least one unaffiliated member ("community member") who can represent community perspectives. Often this is a layperson, such as a member of the clergy.

The federal government designed IRBs to be local committees specifically so that they would represent local community interests and standards. This means that a study approved in Dallas might not receive approval in Boston or Seattle. The idea of local review and oversight is that knowledge of local patient populations, local resources, and the skills and experience of local researchers are to be taken into account when the IRB reviews a protocol.

WHAT DOES THE IRB DO?

The top priority of an IRB is human subject protection. Sometimes this can seem at odds with investigator priorities, which also may include curing disease, adding publications to a curriculum vitae, or supplementing a salary to please a department chair. Institutional review board members (most of whom are faculty researchers themselves) generally think those things are important, too. But their primary focus during IRB review is the protection of human subjects.

Toward that end, IRBs are charged with upholding and enforcing all applicable human subject protection requirements: federal, state, and local. As noted previously, the DHHS regulations known as The Common Rule are the primary regulations for protection of human subjects. In addition, the U.S. Food and Drug Administration (FDA) regulations at 21 CFR Part 56 govern drug and device experimentation, and regulations promulgated by the DHHS Office of Civil Rights protect subject privacy (Health Insurance Portability and Accountability Act, HIPAA). In addition, each state has its own research-related statutes, and all universities and hospitals have research policies and procedures. Institutional review boards must know and adhere to all of these. Ideally, IRBs help investigators understand and comply with these requirements as well.

WHAT DOES THE IRB NEED TO REVIEW?: FOUR KEY POINTS

When deciding whether an activity requires IRB review, it is helpful to parse the federal definition of human research.

1. Is the activity systematic? A case report of one patient who had an unusual drug reaction can be written up, submitted to a journal, and published, but it is not a "systematic investigation ... designed to develop or contribute to generalizable knowledge" (1). By contrast, the deliberate review of multiple case reports in order to generalize the results would constitute a systematic investigation.

2. What is the intent of the investigation? To be considered research, an activity has to be designed in order to develop or contribute to generalizable knowledge. A systematic investigation that involves humans for a purpose other than generating scholarship does not require IRB review. For example, if someone were to undertake a systematic survey asking every third visitor to an office whether the receptionist smiled at them, and if the reason for doing so is to give the receptionist feedback in an annual performance evaluation, then IRB review is not required. However, if the purpose is to write up a paper for a human resources journal about the general level of satisfaction with receptionist friendliness in university administration offices, such a project would need IRB review. For IRB review to be required, it is not necessary to actually make a scholarly contribution but merely to have scholarly intent. Even if an experiment fails or a manuscript never gets published, the time to ask for IRB review is before starting an experiment, if the intention is a research purpose.

3. Are the people under study alive? The federal definition of research covers living humans—not decedents. However, if your research requires collecting data about living humans who are related to the decedents under study, or if you are doing a genetic study that gives you information about the decedents' offspring and such data will be used in the research, the project becomes human research subject by the federal definition. Be careful about knowing your state law on this issue. Most states do not treat research on decedents as human research. However, some states, such as California, have passed laws making research on decedent data and use of cadaveric tissue human research for purposes of IRB oversight.

4. Is the information identifiable? By identifiable, we mean whether the research team has access to identifiers at the time of data collection. For example, a retrospective review of medical charts is human research, even if the researcher does not collect the identifiers for purposes of the study. On the other hand, data that already have been aggregated or deidentified, meaning no individual respondent-level information is available to the researchers (although the information is about living humans), do not meet the federal definition of human subjects research.

In summary, if your investigation is systematic, is done with scholarly intent, and uses humans or identifiable information about living humans, your project meets the federal definition of human subjects research and requires some degree of IRB oversight.

LEVELS OF IRB REVIEW

There are different levels of IRB review depending on the degree of risk posed by a given research study. Investigators need to consider what category of review is appropriate in order to prepare the IRB application. Depending on the research design and the population to be studied, a protocol may qualify for "exemption" from IRB review, for an "expedited" IRB review (which means IRB review by a subcommittee), or for a full-board (i.e., convened meeting) IRB review. Institutional review boards usually have knowledgeable staff that can help investigators to make that determination.

Exempt

"Exempt" means that actual IRB approval is not federally required; however, most institutions require a written validation of exempt status. Usually, verification of exemption is a very simple process. There are six categories of exempt human research defined by regulation, all of which involve virtually no risk to subjects. Examples include retrospective chart reviews when identifiers will not be collected by the researchers, studies of existing deidentified medical specimens, surveys and questionnaires on nonsensitive topics, and taste tests. Verbal consent is appropriate for most kinds of exempt studies, and in many cases, a waiver of consent may be granted.

Expedited

The next level of review is called "expedited." Although this term makes it sound like the review happens extra quickly, in this context, "expedited" simply means the review is performed by a subcommittee of the IRB, rather than by the full board at a convened meeting. According to regulation, to qualify for the expedited subcommittee review, these studies can pose "no more than minimal risk" (1) to subjects, which means no more than the risks of everyday life or a routine medical or psychological examination. For example, a routine medical examination might include measurement of height, weight, blood pressure, some blood work, and urinalysis, but not inoculation with an experimental vaccine. Like the exempt level, there are federally defined categories for expedited review. Written consent often is required, but can be waived by the IRB. Investigators frequently are given permission to obtain verbal consent for expedited studies because they pose no more than minimal risk. The IRB must perform a continuing review of expedited studies at least annually.

Full-Board Review

If a study does not qualify for exemption or expedited review, it must be reviewed at a convened meeting of the full board. These studies involve more than minimal risk to subjects, meaning the risks are higher than those we normally encounter in our everyday lives or at routine medical or psychological examinations. Written consent is required for almost all full-board studies, although there are provisions for waiving consent in some circumstances. Again, continuing review is required at least annually. If an IRB has specific concerns about the safety of a particular study, it can mandate continuing reviews more frequently, such as every six months, each quarter, or after a certain number of subjects is enrolled.

APPLYING FOR IRB REVIEW

Submitting a protocol to the IRB for review requires familiarity with local IRB procedures. At most institutions, the IRB will have a website with application forms and instructions for completing them. Customarily, there is an application form or cover sheet that must be completed by the principal investigator (PI) to initiate the review. That form usually is accompanied by a concise summary of the project (some IRBs call this the "protocol narrative"), an informed consent document (unless requesting a waiver of informed consent), a HIPAA waiver and/or authorization (if needed), and the master protocol and investigator's brochure (these are provided by the pharmaceutical company if it is a clinical trial performed under a contract with a sponsor). If the study is investigator initiated, there usually will not be a master protocol. **Table 2-1** illustrates an example of a checklist that can be used when preparing an IRB application.

THE IRB REVIEW

Once a protocol application comes to the IRB for review, a number of considerations are made by the members.

First, the panel will consider whether the study design is consistent with sound research principles and ethical norms. Although IRBs are not expected to assess scientific merit like study sections, they are charged with assuring a favorable risk-to-benefit ratio. If a scientific design appears so fundamentally flawed that meaningful results will not be possible, the IRB will not be able to justify authorizing even the most modest risks or inconveniences to subjects. The burden is on the PI to explain his/her proposed study design in a way that will show it is possible to answer an important scientific question.

Next, the IRB will determine whether the potential benefits are maximized and the anticipated risks are minimized. In other words, if the study involves a known risk, are there plans to monitor, limit, reverse, or otherwise mitigate it? For example, if a study involves administration of a drug that causes dizziness, will subjects be given a place to lie down or taxi vouchers so they do not try to drive themselves home?

Similarly, if a study benefit can be maximized, there should be plans to do so. A common way to maximize benefits for study subjects is to share with them information relevant to their medical care. If the study involves testing for disease prevalence in a population, the IRB may ask whether plans have been made to refer subjects for treatment in the event of a clinically relevant finding.

Another important consideration made by the IRB is whether the plan for selection of study subjects appears equitable. One of the pillars of human subject protection is the

TABLE **2-1** | Checklist for Use in Preparation of an IRB Protocol Submission

Step	Description
1.	Make sure that all study personnel have been trained on human subject protection requirements in accordance with local IRB policy. Often the required training is available online. Consult your local IRB to find out if collaborators outside your institution need to take your local IRB training in order to be listed on a protocol application.
2.	Be certain that all the required components are included in the submission packet. Protocol reviews frequently are delayed simply because the packet is missing an essential document, such as an informed consent form or a master protocol.
3.	Provide enough information to the IRB so that they can make a decision. This is especially true when proposing a study that is controversial or ethically provocative. If the study is likely to raise IRB "eyebrows," be proactive about providing a rationale in terms the IRB members can understand. For example, when reviewing a placebo-controlled trial of a new drug to treat a disorder for which there is a safe and efficacious treatment already on the market, the IRB will want to know that thought has been given to whether it is ethical to deny treatment to the control arm for the duration of the study, and why the benefit of this study outweighs the risk to those individuals who go untreated during the trial. Similarly, if a study is designed to obtain informed consent from women who are in active labor, the IRB will want an explanation of why the research cannot be done in some other population that is not in pain and under duress. If it appears to the IRB members that there is not a well thought-out reason for conducting an ethically provocative study, they are likely to defer the application pending further dialogue with the investigator.
4.	Avoid unnecessary jargon and abbreviations. This is important not only because it is hard for the scientific members to review a protocol in another scientific discipline, but—more importantly—it is critical for the unaffiliated "community members" sitting on these boards. If you give a highly technical explanation of the proposed study, laypeople sitting on the IRB simply may not be able to understand it. Keeping the protocol documents relatively free of jargon greatly facilitates the review process.
5.	Double-check grammar, syntax, spelling, and formatting. Ask a colleague to proofread the drafts. Scientists frequently criticize the IRB for nitpicking spelling but IRB members often have two kinds of legitimate concerns when sloppy documents are submitted for review. First, when asking the IRB to authorize an experiment on humans, it should be evident that sufficient thought and attention have gone into the study proposal. When an investigator cannot be bothered even to run a spell-checker, it suggests s/he is not giving the project adequate attention. Second, it is important to note that occasionally typographical errors really matter. The difference between "by month" and "by mouth" in an informed consent document is both substantive and important to subject safety.

RESEARCH ETHICS: PITFALLS & PRESCRIPTIONS

Reasonable people can disagree about ethical issues, and IRBs and clinical investigators are no exception. When investigators have ethical concerns about any aspects of their protocols, an early phone call or visit with an IRB staff member often can clarify matters and avoid unnecessary disagreements or delays. Moreover, following the National Institutes of Health Clinical Translational Science Initiative, many academic medical centers have developed research ethics consultation services that can offer ethics assistance and advice at any stage of a protocol's development and execution. Investigators should recognize that the IRB's primary role is protection of research participants' rights and welfare; ethical problems in other stages or domains of research may not be addressed by the IRB. These may include, for example, authorship disputes, unanticipated ethical dilemmas arising in the conduct of the trial, or issues in submission and publication of research.

Beskow LM, Grady C, Iltis AS, et al. Points to consider: The research ethics consultation service and the IRB. *IRB*. 2009;31(6):1–9.

principle of justice. This means that we ought not burden vulnerable populations unduly nor reserve the benefits of research only for the very privileged. Institutional review board members will review the recruitment plan and will raise questions about who may be targeted specifically or left out (whether intentionally or by default).

Institutional review boards also must evaluate whether all the necessary elements of informed consent have been included in the consent form that will be given to subjects. The required consent elements are listed in *The Common Rule* and most research institutions host a link to them on the website of the local IRB. Some IRBs also have an informed consent template that researchers can use to help prevent leaving out a required element while drafting the consent document.

Protection of subject privacy is another important issue considered by the IRB. The study plan will be scrutinized to assure that all necessary precautions are in place to protect subject privacy and to preserve confidentiality of study data. In this age of rapidly changing technology, procedures for data collection and storage have become highly complex. It is important to explain not only where hard copies of paper consent forms will be kept under lock and key, but also what schemes will be used for encryption of digital data, firewall protection of computers, and even how hackers will be prevented for intercepting data collection and transmission using web portals, handheld (mobile) devices, or remote sensors.

Finally, IRBs are mandated to consider whether additional safeguards are in place to protect especially vulnerable subject populations. For example, if children will be studied, there must be a plan for obtaining parental permission. It also may be appropriate to seek assent from the minor subjects. Similarly, the study of decisionally impaired people usually requires plans to obtain consent from the subjects' legally authorized representatives. Other categories of special populations requiring extra protections include prisoners, pregnant women and fetuses, and subordinate employees of the researcher.

OF SPECIAL CONCERN TO IRBs

Beyond the extra protections required for vulnerable subject populations, IRBs frequently are concerned about other special topics related to human subject protection.

Show Me the Money

Research risks are not only physical; they also can be emotional, and even financial. If a researcher proposes to bill subjects for the experimental drug or device under study, the IRB members will want to know why. Is there a reason that the company sponsoring the trial is not providing their product free to subjects? Sometimes billing subjects or insurers for study-related expenses can be appropriate, such as in cancer cooperative group trials comparing two accepted standards of care, but it is important to provide a justification.

Exclusion of Non-English Speakers

Regulations require that informed consent is documented in a language understandable to the subject. Unless written consent is waived, that means getting it translated in writing into the language(s) that the likely subjects speak. This concern relates to the question of whether the distribution of risks and benefits in society is equitable. An IRB will not likely be sympathetic to a statement like, "Non-English speakers will be excluded because we do not want to spend money to translate the consent form." However, there can be legitimate scientific reasons for language exclusions. For example, "We must exclude non-English speakers from this psychiatric study because the data collection instruments have not been validated in any language other than English."

Off-Site Research

Researchers proposing to conduct experiments outside their institution of employment should expect to provide extra documentation. Frequently, an IRB will require evidence that the proposed off-site study locations have given permission to conduct research on their premises. If the off-site institution(s) has an IRB, chances are that their IRB also will want to review the study before the work begins at that site. Consultation with your local IRB about requirements for authorization of off-site research can save a lot of time.

Drugs, Devices, and Biologics

The FDA regulates experiments using new drugs, devices, and biologics by issuing permission to use Investigational New Drugs and through Investigational Device Exemptions. Frequently, investigators want to test an existing drug for a new indication. That also sometimes needs an Investigational New Drug, so it is important to consult with your local IRB whenever planning a study that involves the use of drugs. When a clinical trial is sponsored by industry (whether a pharmaceutical company or a device manufacturer), chances are they already obtained FDA permission for the trial before recruiting investigators. This is something the PI should verify before applying for IRB approval locally. This topic is described in more detail in Chapter 11.

RESEARCH ETHICS: PITFALLS & PRESCRIPTIONS

Biotechnology is advancing at an extraordinary rate, and at the time of this writing, the FDA is revising its regulations to address new technologies that may not be addressed adequately by the current regulations. For instance, nanodevices and nanoparticles are being developed to deliver drugs to specific sites in the body. Should these be considered drugs, devices, both, or neither? Investigators working with emerging technologies should consult their IRB (and in some cases the FDA offices directly) before proceeding to help identify novel ethical issues as well as address the applicability of the regulations.

Wilson RF. Nanotechnology: the challenge of regulating known unknowns. Symposium article. *J Law Med Ethics*. 2006;34:704–713.

Health Insurance Portability and Accountability Act

This relatively new law affects research involving the creation, use, or sharing of identifiable health information. At many academic medical centers and hospitals, the IRB acts as the "privacy committee" required by HIPAA, meaning that it reviews the plans for protecting private information about patients. Depending on the study design, you may need to provide a HIPAA authorization and/or a HIPAA waiver request to your IRB with the application to conduct human research. The HIPAA waiver is a document that allows a researcher to access people's private information without their knowledge or permission. For example, if a PI wants to review 500 medical charts of people with a certain diagnosis, she/he would need permission from the IRB to conduct the study and also would need a HIPAA waiver to look at the charts without getting permission from the patients themselves. A HIPAA authorization is different. A HIPAA authorization is something that a PI will use to get permission from the study subjects to access their private health information or to transmit their private information to another entity. For clinical trials, subjects typically sign both the research-informed consent form and a HIPAA authorization permitting use of their health information for the study. At some institutions, the HIPAA authorization language is integrated into the research-informed consent document; however, some states have laws that prohibit this. This topic is discussed in detail in Chapters 3 and 4.

Certificates of Confidentiality

When a study involves collection of information that is potentially stigmatizing (e.g., could put someone at risk for legal prosecution, being fired, getting deported, or put on the news and shunned by their friends and neighbors), the IRB may ask an investigator to apply for a certificate of confidentiality from the National Institutes of Health (NIH). This document protects an investigator from having to disclose any research-related information to a requestor, even under a subpoena. For example, if a subject is in the middle of divorce proceedings, and the PI of the study gets a subpoena from the husband's attorney requesting study records to see if the wife disclosed drug use on a study questionnaire, a certificate of confidentiality would allow the PI to respond, "I'm sorry. I can't even confirm that person was in this study. I have a certificate of confidentiality from NIH."

Genetic Testing

Protocols involving the use of genetic tests get extra scrutiny from IRBs for several reasons. One major concern is the possibility that the information derived can place subjects at risk for discrimination by employers and health or life insurance companies (accordingly, the IRB may recommend a certificate of confidentiality). Another issue is the psychological distress that may be experienced by subjects who learn of a genetic predisposition to develop a disease. In addition, genetic studies sometimes can yield unexpected findings, such as misattributed paternity. For these and other reasons, many IRBs require additional consent language to inform subjects about the particular risks associated with genetic testing. Some IRBs even require the use of separate genetic research consent forms or consent form appendices to address these concerns in greater detail (see Chapters 3 and 4).

COMMON REASONS FOR IRB DELAYS

Institutional review board approval can be delayed for any number of reasons. Keep in mind that the IRB staff members whose job is to write those IRB determination memos are just the messengers. The voting members who sit on the boards—your colleagues— make the decisions. Although it might feel really good to yell at the IRB staff when you do not like an IRB decision, it does not actually result in your protocol getting approved any faster. To help you avoid common pitfalls, a list of the top 10 reasons for IRB delays is illustrated in **Table 2-2**.

Study Management

Once you have IRB approval, regulations and requirements that affect the conduct of the study must be followed. From the perspective of the IRB, these are the most important things to keep in mind.

Recruitment

One thing that often is not understood is that recruitment is the beginning of the informed consent process. For this reason, the IRB must approve the text of any poster, classified ad, radio spot, e-mail message, or television commercial used to recruit study subjects.

If you place an advertisement in the newspaper or put flyers up around a campus to interest people in your study, it is really important that the ads are not misleading. This is especially of concern when recruiting for clinical trials of drugs and devices because the FDA has specific requirements for what can (and cannot) be said in a study recruitment ad.

Overemphasizing financial inducements may cause potential subjects to consider the reward first and the potential risks later. For this reason, an ad that says, "FREE HEALTH CARE! FREE DRUGS! EARN $500 TODAY!" in all capital letters, bolded, and underlined will be perceived by the IRB as undue pressure and would not likely be approved.

Keep in mind that the methods of advertising proposed in the recruitment section of your protocol narrative are the ones the IRB expects you to use. If you find that the recruitment strategy that you originally proposed is not working and you are not able to accrue

TABLE **2-2** | Common Reasons for IRB Delays

1. Research team members have not completed required human subjects protection training.

2. Required signatures or authorizations are missing. Most IRBs require a signature (electronic or hard copy) from the lead researcher and some sort of permission or concurrence from his/her department chair or supervisor.

3. Research is to be conducted off-site and evidence of permission from the off-site institution is not provided.

4. Protocol requires review by another institutional entity. At most institutions, the IRB is one of many review bodies that must authorize a study before it can begin. For example, if the protocol is cancer-related (which includes cancer prevention, cancer treatment, cancer survival, or even quality of life for cancer survivors), review by the protocol review and monitoring committee of the cancer center usually is required before the study can be approved by the IRB. Similarly, if the study involves radiation (e.g., x-rays and positron emission tomography scans), approval from the radiation use committee may be required.

5. Significant discrepancies between the protocol and consent form. Institutional review board members review the documents submitted by the PI carefully. If the protocol says there is a risk of hair loss, dizziness, and occasionally death but the consent form lists only the risk of occasional hair loss, the IRB will ask the investigator for revisions to ensure consistency.

6. Recruitment procedures and informed consent process not adequately explained. It is not enough to simply request 100 subjects. The methods of recruitment and sources of subjects are important, too. Tell the IRB if you plan to recruit from among your own patients or from an online chat room for potential participants. The "how" is as important as the "who."

7. Anticipated risks to the participants not justified. Although it is perfectly acceptable to propose procedures that are risky for subjects, there must be corresponding benefits for subjects and/or for society. A rationale for the known risks must be provided in the protocol.

8. Inadequate safeguards to protect data from a breach of confidentiality. If the safeguards are not sufficient, the IRB will ask for more information to assure that risks associated with unauthorized access to subjects' data are minimized to the fullest extent possible.

9. Consent form deficient. If the consent form is missing required elements, or if the reading level is too high or contains too much jargon, the IRB will ask for revisions.

10. No scientific justification for exclusion of non-English speakers or no description of plan to enroll non-English speakers. In some parts of the country, this is not a frequent IRB concern. However, in most urban areas and in all of the southwest, IRBs pay great attention to language issues both because of the potential for inadvertent exclusion of otherwise eligible subjects and because of the requirement that consent be understandable to subjects.

subjects as quickly as you wanted, then you need to submit a modification request to the IRB saying that you would like to change methods for recruitment and describing the proposed changes.

Enrollment

Consent is a process, not a document. Although the IRB scrutinizes the informed consent form to make sure it contains all the required elements, the paper form is meant to memorialize the fact that a dialogue took place between researcher and subject about the risks and benefits of participation. Signing the form is a formality that should follow a verbal invitation, a thorough explanation of the facts, and an opportunity for the subject to ask questions and consider without pressure whether or not to enroll.

Keep in mind that once the informed consent form is approved by the IRB, the approved form is the only version you should use to document the willingness of a subject to participate in the research project. Some investigators will photocopy the original version approved by the IRB. Others will scan it and host it on a shared drive so that other people on the study team can download it and print it off. Either way is acceptable, but it is essential to use the approved version. Do not alter or add to an IRB-approved informed consent form.

Modifications

Any change to an approved study must be approved by the IRB before you make that change. This includes adding a new member to the study team, changing study procedures, changing subject populations, and adding recruitment methods. Most IRBs have a form for requesting permission to modify a study. In rare circumstances, a PI may alter a study procedure to avoid an immediate apparent hazard to a subject without prior IRB permission; however, these deviations should be reported to the IRB as soon as possible.

There are two kinds of IRB modifications. A minor change can be reviewed via the expedited method (i.e., by subcommittee). Any significant change (one that affects the risk–benefit ratio or substantially changes what the study is trying to accomplish) must be reviewed by the full board at a convened meeting. Sometimes an IRB will determine that significant changes resulting in new informed consent language warrant "reconsenting" of already enrolled subjects because the new information may affect their willingness to continue participating.

It is the significance of the modification itself that affects whether it goes to full board or is expedited, not the initial level of review of the study. Therefore, a significant change to an expedited study could still go to the full board. Likewise, a minor change to a full-board study can be reviewed via the expedited procedure. Frequently, significant changes to expedited studies cause them to become full-board studies.

Adverse Events and Unanticipated Problems

Any time something happens to a subject that is not good and that was unexpected (i.e., not identified as a known risk in the informed consent document), the incident must be reported to the IRB. Many IRBs have an "Adverse Event" (AE) form for this purpose. The most serious AEs (called SAEs), which are death, hospitalization, prolongation of a planned hospitalization, and birth defects, need to be reported to the IRB immediately—preferably by phone or fax—and followed by a written report.

Even events that do not appear to be related to the study intervention are reportable. Some investigators may assume, for example, that a broken arm need not be reported because it does not appear to be a study-related injury. However, seemingly unrelated events can signal new, previously unknown risks. If five subjects on a trial break limbs in a one-month period, it may suggest that the study drug causes dizziness. Only if these events are reported can the IRB do the type of trend analyses that can identify new risk information. Such information is vital, not only because it informs the IRB's decision about permitting the study to continue, but also because it is essential for keeping the informed consent document complete and up-to-date.

The IRB takes into account the health of the subjects when it reviews AE reports. Studies including sick populations will be expected to report multiple hospitalizations and even deaths. However, a study of healthy volunteers with lots of unanticipated hospitalizations will raise red flags.

It should be noted that the IRB is not a Data Safety and Monitoring Board (DSMB), and it may have difficulty interpreting AE data for a multisite study sponsored by a pharmaceutical company. Local IRBs only have complete information about subjects enrolled on-site, so they must rely on the sponsor monitors and the national (or international) DSMB to provide a more rigorous review, inclusive of study-wide data. Institutional review boards expect that a local PI will provide DSMB reports as they are forwarded by the study sponsor or at least at the time of continuing review. These reports complement the AE reports already received in the IRB office by providing a context based on study-wide analyses.

Deviations and Violations

These two words often are used interchangeably to describe a variance from approved study procedures or timelines. An examination of 10 IRB websites at 10 universities across the country will reveal 20 different definitions of the words "deviation" and "violation." Some IRBs only use one word, some use only the other word, and some use both words and distinguish between them. The bottom line is that altering the approved protocol without prior IRB approval of a modification should be unusual and must be justified and documented.

For example, if a study subject is supposed to have laboratory tests on day 14 but unexpectedly has to leave town to attend a funeral and makes arrangements to have the tests performed on day 22, this is a variance from the protocol. An investigator may consider this as a minor difference as to be irrelevant. However, a study sponsor may disqualify the subject and disregard their data. The IRB may consider an alteration to the study schedule noncompliance with the protocol. For this reason, it is important to communicate with the sponsor and the IRB when a protocol deviation or violation occurs.

Many times the sponsor will want to "preauthorize" a deviation and may give you permission over the phone or by fax for a variance from their protocol. Investigators should understand that approval of a study deviation by a trial sponsor does not take the place of IRB approval of a change in your protocol. Such events need to be reported to the IRB. In fact, when a study sponsor approves a deviation, they usually want to see proof that the variance is acceptable to the IRB. Most investigators find that if they forward the sponsor's authorization for a one-time variance to the IRB, obtaining documentation of IRB acknowledgement can be relatively straightforward. An IRB chair may ask the investigator whether a modification of the protocol is warranted, and the investigator should be prepared to explain whether the circumstances at hand are likely to happen again with sufficient frequency as to suggest a modification is appropriate.

Communicating with Sponsors

Investigators should be aware that when they agree to conduct a clinical trial paid for by a private company, that company will have its own idiosyncratic procedures and its own bureaucratic jargon. Sometimes the sponsor will host a meeting to kick off a study, often in a really nice place. At this meeting, the sponsor will explain its expectations, including preferences about how they want investigators to communicate with them. It is really important to foster a good relationship with the sponsor. Decide early in the study who on your team is the designated point of contact with the sponsor and channel all communications through him/her. It is best to keep a notebook of all communications with the trial sponsor. When communicating with the sponsor by phone, document who was on the call, what was said, and when the call took place. E-mail can be handy because it is already date-stamped, and it shows who sent and received the message. Print e-mails out and file them in the study notebook. The purpose of documentation is to avoid a scenario in which the sponsor authorizes a deviation by phone and you have no evidence to prove it to the IRB or the FDA.

Retain all study-related records and be prepared to show source documents. The sponsor may want to come on site periodically and look at your recordkeeping to compare your case report forms to the source documents. It can be very helpful to perform self-assessment audits periodically to make sure, for example, that the laboratory values in the patient chart match what you have recorded on the case report form.

Anything the sponsor tells you about how well (or not well) you are meeting regulatory obligations is something you should share with the IRB. If the sponsor does an on-site audit and issues a report, even if it is a clean bill of health, the documents relating to the visit should be forwarded to the IRB. In like fashion, a report that documents that "In three cases, the PI failed to sign the consent document and did not attach a HIPAA authorization," also should be sent to the IRB.

Continuing Review

When the IRB approves a protocol, they give permission to conduct the trial for an interval of time. Usually a trial is approved for 365 days from the review date. Keep in mind that the review date may not be the same as the approval date. For example, if your protocol is reviewed in November, but you do not respond to the IRB stipulations until January, the approval date will be in January, although the anniversary of the review will be in November. The protocol approval expires the day before the year anniversary of the review date, not the approval date. Using the example previously mentioned, if your protocol is reviewed on November 1 and your approval letter is dated January 14, approval will expire on October 31.

Remember that the IRB has the authority to approve a protocol for a period less than 365 days. If the committee members believe that the intervention is especially risky, if the committee is concerned that an especially vulnerable subject population is involved that needs closer oversight, or if the trial involves very sensitive issues, the IRB may approve a protocol for only 6 months. In such instances, the IRB may grant approval for enrollment of a limited number of subjects and require rereview before approving the enrollment of additional participants. Because the interval of approval is decided by the IRB and can be shorter than 1 year, it is important to pay attention to what the approval letter says.

Assuming normal circumstances, the project approval will be valid for 365 days from the date of review. Most IRBs will send a reminder memo before expiration of the protocol approval that says something like, "Your protocol approval for study XYZ is going to expire on such-and-such date, we recommend you submit your continuing review application documents ASAP." This is important because if your study approval lapses, you will be out of compliance with the federal oversight regulations. You will make your sponsor very unhappy, and—if your sponsor happens to be the federal government—they will prohibit you from spending grant funds during the period of lapsed IRB approval.

Many IRBs have a form that needs to be filled out to request a continuing review. That form captures information such as how many subjects were enrolled during the last performance period, whether there were adverse events, and whether there will be any changes in procedures or study personnel over the coming year. If the study is a multisite trial, often there will be a DSMB. If the DSMB has issued an interim report, it should be provided to the IRB at continuing review. So, get your continuing review request in before your study approval expires, write a brief but informative progress report, locate and attach any DSMB reports that may have been forwarded to you by the sponsor. If the study is a cooperative group trial, this may come from the cooperative group coordinating board, or whoever is assigned to do data safety monitoring. Be prepared to justify either no or slow enrollment, high dropout rate, or excessive complaints or problems.

Continuing review is not a "rubber stamp" process. The regulations require it to be a substantive review. It gives the IRB the opportunity to reevaluate the importance of the research question and the appropriateness of the risks, to analyze the adverse events, and to look at any potential need to modify the protocol or the consent. Although the IRB is not a scientific review panel, the IRB will look at the importance of the research question in the context of performing an analysis of the risks-to-benefit ratio. If a study began in 1980, and it is still ongoing in 2008, the IRB may perform a literature review on your hypothesis and find that six other teams around the world have definitively answered this question already. In such a case, repeating the experiment now would be of very little benefit. In such a case, the IRB may ask for a justification for exposing subjects to the research risks.

Although not usually the case, it is possible at continuing review for the IRB to require changes that are different than what the first board said at the time of initial approval. Each board consists of human beings and, by nature, human beings are idiosyncratic. The initial review board can approve a study the first time, and then at the next continuing review can identify new problems. Investigators should not be surprised to receive legitimate critiques or requests for changes from year to year.

POSTAPPROVAL MONITORING

In addition to the routine continuing review that the IRB performs at board meetings, most IRBs also do some kind of "not-for-cause" (routine) postapproval monitoring where staff members are sent to make certain that approved protocols have been followed and all elements of a study are well documented.

Institutional review boards also conduct audits for cause in the event of a complaint, allegation, or safety concern. It might be a parent upset that his child never got paid for participation in a study. It could be an adult on a placebo-controlled trial who feels that her problem is getting worse, and she is afraid to tell the investigator because she does not want to disappoint her physician. It could be people who feel that they were unfairly screened out of a study to which they believe they deserved access.

The FDA also audits periodically. The FDA usually conducts their audits at the point when they are about to take a new drug or device to market. They want to go back and look at the data at each of the sites to make sure that the data are good before they take that next step. If the FDA comes to do an audit, the investigator should always ask to see a badge. If you do not ask to see a badge, they will write you up for noncompliance. It is not only your right to ask to see FDA identification; it is your obligation. Otherwise, you may be releasing proprietary information of the sponsor or you may be releasing subject identifying information to an unauthorized person. In such circumstances, it is important to tell your IRB if the FDA comes to conduct an audit. The IRB can assist by sitting in and answering any questions the FDA inspector may have.

Although most of the time researchers do their best to comply with all the rules, sometimes mistakes are made. When an error is inadvertent and does not appear to affect subject safety or welfare, an IRB usually will try to resolve it informally. Occasionally, IRBs encounter investigators who deliberately break a rule, willfully disregard IRB procedure, or behave unethically. Most IRBs have procedures for handling allegations of regulatory noncompliance. Often, the process begins with an administrative review. This means pulling the protocol file to see what was approved. Sometimes allegations can be dismissed right away simply by reviewing the record.

When informal resolution is not possible, the IRB does have the authority to impose corrective action. In response to concerns about noncompliance, IRBs may restrict protocol approvals to intervals shorter that 1 year. They can require that a PI have a "proctor" to oversee their work. The IRB also can suspend or terminate protocol approvals, which must be reported to the federal regulatory authorities, including the funding agencies (a truly undesirable outcome). In extreme cases, a PI can be told, "Doing research is a privilege, and you have just lost the privilege." This sometimes is called the "death penalty." Beyond the restrictions that may be imposed by the IRB, universities and hospitals also can impose penalties for research noncompliance. There can be additional remedies that involve placement of letters in a personnel file, demotion, sending a retraction letter to a journal, and a number of other corrective actions.

CLOSING A PROTOCOL

At the end of a study, investigators should close out the protocol with their local IRB. Keep in mind that if there is a reasonable chance access to the identifiable private information will be needed again, the protocol should remain open. However, when analyses of identifiable data are complete, it is best to close it out. For the most part, the local IRB is required to keep its records from three to six years following study closure.

RESEARCH ETHICS: PITFALLS & PRESCRIPTIONS

Related to study closure is the ethical problem of abandoning studies. Abandoning a study means that the investigator or research team has discontinued the conduct of the research without completing the protocol. Abandoning studies can be unethical because it usually means the scientific benefits of the study are not realized; therefore, the risks that study participants have undergone are not justified. Moreover, abandoning a study may inappropriately place responsibility on others (junior investigator, secretary, etc.) who are poorly qualified to conduct or complete the research, putting participants at additional risk. This problem can occur for multiple reasons (death/serious illness of the investigator, accepting a new job elsewhere, etc.). Studies should always be closed or transferred officially through the IRB office.

CONCLUSIONS

In summary, the various regulatory requirements for clinical research are complicated and can be daunting. However, local IRBs usually have trained and capable personnel who can help investigators to navigate the gauntlet of forms, reports, and other obligations. In moments of frustration, it is important to keep in mind that good treatment of research subjects yields good science. Finally, the protection of human research subjects' rights and welfare is not only the right thing to do—it is the law.

REFERENCE

1. Code of Federal Regulations, Title 45, Part 46. Protection of Human Subjects. Revised June 23, 2005.

CHAPTER 3

Writing Informed Consent Documents and Obtaining Informed Consent

Anne Clark, CIP, Suzanne M. Rivera, PhD, MSW, P. Diane Sheppard, RN, Darren K. McGuire, MD, MHSc, and Michael J. McPhaul, MD

OUTLINE

Introduction

Belmont Commission

Code of Federal Regulations

Required Elements

Required element 1—the research declaration

Required element 2—identification of foreseeable risks or discomforts

Required element 3—identification of possible benefits

Required element 4—alternatives to participation

Required element 5—confidentiality

Required element 6—compensation

Required element 7—contact Information

Required element 8—participation is voluntary

Additional Elements

Guidelines for Preparing Consent Forms and Assuring an Effective and Valid Consenting Process

Documentation of Informed Consent

What Activities Are Subject to IRB Review?

Waivers and Alterations of Informed Consent

Waiver of Documentation of Informed Consent (Verbal Consent)

Non-English-Speaking Subjects and Translation of Consent Documents

DNA and Unused Samples

HIPAA Authorization and Waiver of Authorizations

HIPAA Waiver of Authorization

The Process of Obtaining Informed Consent

INTRODUCTION

For many people today, human research subject protection requirements like formal IRB study protocols and informed consent documents are part of the fabric of clinical investigation. However, the concept of ethical oversight of human investigation is only about 65 years old and formal consent documents have only been required for clinical research in the United States for about 30 years.

TABLE **3-1** | **Nuremberg Code**

1. The voluntary consent of the human subject is absolutely essential. This means that the person involved should have legal capacity to give consent; should be so situated as to be able to exercise free power of choice, without the intervention of any element of force, fraud, deceit, duress, over-reaching, or other ulterior form of constraint or coercion; and should have sufficient knowledge and comprehension of the elements of the subject matter involved as to enable him to make an understanding and enlightened decision. This latter element requires that before the acceptance of an affirmative decision by the experimental subject, it should be made known to him the nature, duration, and purpose of the experiment; the method and means by which it is to be conducted; and all inconveniences and hazards reasonable to be expected; and the effects upon his health or person, which may possibly come from his participation in the experiment. The duty and responsibility for ascertaining the quality of the consent rests upon each individual who initiates, directs, or engages in the experiment. It is a personal duty and responsibility that may not be delegated to another with impunity.

2. The experiment should be such as to yield fruitful results for the good of society, unprocurable by other methods or means of study, and not random and unnecessary in nature.

3. The experiment should be so designed and based on the results of animal experimentation and knowledge of the natural history of the disease or other problem under study that the anticipated results will justify the performance of the experiment.

4. The experiment should be so conducted as to avoid all unnecessary physical and mental suffering and injury.

5. No experiment should be conducted where there is an a priori reason to believe that death or disabling injury will occur, except, perhaps, in those experiments where the experimental physicians also serve as subjects.

6. The degree of risk to be taken should never exceed that determined by the humanitarian importance of the problem to be solved by the experiment.

7. Proper preparations should be made and adequate facilities provided to protect the experimental subject against even remote possibilities of injury, disability, or death.

8. The experiment should be conducted only by scientifically qualified persons. The highest degree of skill and care should be required through all stages of the experiment of those who conduct or engage in the experiment.

9. During the course of the experiment, the human subject should be at liberty to bring the experiment to an end if he has reached the physical or mental state where continuation of the experiment seems to him to be impossible.

10. During the course of the experiment, the scientist in charge must be prepared to terminate the experiment at any stage, if he has probable cause to believe, in the exercise of the good faith, superior skill, and careful judgment required of him that a continuation of the experiment is likely to result in injury, disability, or death to the experimental subject.

(http://ohsr.od.nih.gov/guidelines/nuremberg.html)

T A B L E   **3-2** | **Declaration of Helsinki (1964, with Several Subsequent Refinements)**

The basic principles of the Declaration of Helsinki include the following:
- Physician's duty in research is to protect the life, health, privacy, and dignity of the human participant
- Research involving humans must conform to generally accepted scientific principles and thorough knowledge of scientific literature and methods
- Research protocols should be reviewed by an independent committee
- Research protocols should be conducted by medically/scientifically qualified individuals
- Risks and burden to the participant should not outweigh benefits
- Researcher should stop study if risks are found to outweigh potential benefits
- Research is justified only if there is a reasonable likelihood that the population under study will benefit from the results
- Participants must be volunteers and informed in research project
- Every precaution must be taken to respect privacy, confidentiality, and participant's physical and mental integrity
- Assent must be obtained from minors, if a child is able to do so
- Investigators are obliged to preserve the accuracy of results; negative and positive results

Available at World Medical Association website: http://www.wma.net.

A number of landmark events and documents have shaped the regulatory requirements governing the conduct of human research and the need for specific informed consent elements. The first of these were the disclosures and deliberations surrounding the medical experimentation that was conducted by the Nazis during World War II. The revelation of the nature and scope of these activities during the Nuremberg tribunal led to the enumeration of 10 ethical principles for the conduct of human research. **Table 3-1** lists the elements of the Nuremberg Code, which has shaped the perception and conduct of human experimentation in subsequent generations. These elements were refined and restated by the global medical community in 1964 in the Declaration of Helsinki. As is evident from an inspection of **Table 3-2**, many of the tenets established in the Nuremberg Code are restated and refined in the Helsinki Declaration. Although these documents never were codified in law and are not legally binding, they are regarded as cornerstones of human research ethics.

BELMONT COMMISSION

Despite the heightened awareness of the need to protect research participants' rights following dissemination of the Nuremberg Code and the Declaration of Helsinki, revelations of additional research abuses, such as the NIH-funded Tuskegee syphilis study, continued to focus attention on the improper conduct of human research. Against this backdrop, the National Research Act was passed, authorizing the National Commission for the Protection

T A B L E **3-3** | **The Belmont Report, United States (1979)**

On July 12, 1974, the U.S. National Commission for the Protection of Human Subjects of Biomedical and Behavioral Research was created via the U.S. National Research Act. The Commission was to:
- Identify the basic ethical principles that should underlie the conduct of biomedical and behavioral research involving human subjects and
- Develop guidelines that should be followed to assure that biomedical and behavioral research is conducted in accordance with the basic ethical principles.

The basic ethical principles of The Belmont Report (http://www.hhs.gov/ohrp/humansubjects/guidance/belmont.htm) are as follows:
1. Respect for persons
    - Autonomy of individuals
    - Persons with diminished autonomy are entitled to protection
2. Beneficence
    - Respect persons' decisions and protect from harm
    - Maximize possible benefits and minimize possible harms
3. Justice
    - Benefits and risks of research must be distributed fairly
    The applications of 1, 2, and 3, respectively, are informed consent, assessment of risks and benefits, and selection of subjects

http://www.wma.net/e/policy/b3.htm

of Human Subjects of Biomedical and Behavioral Research. One of the principal objectives of this body was to enumerate basic ethical principles to guide the conduct of human research and guidelines that researchers should follow in such activities. The Belmont Report represents the findings of a 4-day conference held in 1976 and subsequent discussions among the Commission members over a 4-year period. These proceedings were published in the Federal Register. The principles informed development of federal regulations that govern the IRB review of research, including elements of informed consent.

The Belmont Report distilled the Nuremberg Code and the Declaration of Helsinki into three overarching ethical principles: autonomy, beneficence, and justice **(Table 3-3)**. First and foremost is respect for persons, also known as autonomy. This is reflected in an individual's decision to accept or refuse participation in research. This is followed by beneficence, defined as benefiting the individual or humankind, while minimizing unnecessary risks. Finally, the research must be just. That is, it must be fair and equitable, neither targeting nor benefiting one group of individuals over another.

CODE OF FEDERAL REGULATIONS

The U.S. regulations governing human research, including informed consent, are listed in the Code of Federal Regulations (CFR), and contain the required elements of informed consent. The U.S. Department of Health and Human Services (DHHS) serves as the oversight

---

RESEARCH ETHICS: PITFALLS & PRESCRIPTIONS

Informed consent requirements represent a community consensus about the kinds of information (and method of delivery) a reasonable person would need to make an informed decision about participation in research. In preparing a study protocol, the investigator should identify and address any ethically challenging consent issues by (1) considering the applicability of each required element of informed consent and (2) customizing the consent forms and processes in the context of the study and the intended subject population(s) to maximize comprehension and free choice.

---

agency with enforcement authority. The regulations (known as 45 CFR 46) outline the basic requirements for protection of human subjects. The specific requirements for informed consent are outlined in Section 116. These include both required and optional elements **(Table 3-4)**. These elements should guide the construction of any informed consent document. Note that these are not recommendations or guidance; they are required in order for a consent document to be considered legally effective.

T A B L E **3-4** | **General Requirements for Informed Consent- Code of Federal Regulations, Title 45, Part 46, Section 116 (45 CFR 46 CFR § 46.116)**

Except as provided elsewhere in this policy, no investigator may involve a human being as a subject in research covered by this policy unless the investigator has obtained the legally effective informed consent of the subject or the subject's legally authorized representative. An investigator shall seek such consent only under circumstances that provide the prospective subject or the representative sufficient opportunity to consider whether or not to participate and that minimize the possibility of coercion or undue influence. The information that is given to the subject or the representative shall be in language understandable to the subject or the representative. No informed consent, whether oral or written, may include any exculpatory language through which the subject or the representative is made to waive or appear to waive any of the subject's legal rights, or releases or appears to release the investigator, the sponsor, the institution, or its agents from liability for negligence.

(a) Basic elements of informed consent. Except as provided in paragraph (c) (http://www.hhs.gov/ohrp/humansubjects/guidance/45cfr46.htm#46.116(c)#46.116(c)) or (d) (http://www.hhs.gov/ohrp/humansubjects/guidance/45cfr46.htm#46.116(d)#46.116(d)) of this section, in seeking informed consent the following information shall be provided to each subject:

(1) A statement that the study involves research, an explanation of the purposes of the research and the expected duration of the subject's participation, a description of the procedures to be followed, and identification of any procedures that are experimental;

(2) A description of any reasonably foreseeable risks or discomforts to the subject;

(3) A description of any benefits to the subject or to others, which may reasonably be expected from the research;

(continued)

TABLE **3-4** | General Requirements for Informed Consent-Code of Federal Regulations, Title 45, Part 46, Section 116 (45 CFR 46 CFR § 46.116) *(continued)*

(4) A disclosure of appropriate alternative procedures or courses of treatment, if any, that might be advantageous to the subject;

(5) A statement describing the extent, if any, to which confidentiality of records identifying the subject will be maintained;

(6) For research involving more than minimal risk, an explanation as to whether any compensation and an explanation as to whether any medical treatments are available if injury occurs and, if so, what they consist of, or where further information may be obtained;

(7) An explanation of whom to contact for answers to pertinent questions about the research and research subjects' rights, and whom to contact in the event of a research-related injury to the subject; and

(8) A statement that participation is voluntary, refusal to participate will involve no penalty or loss of benefits to which the subject is otherwise entitled, and the subject may discontinue participation at any time without penalty or loss of benefits to which the subject is otherwise entitled.

(b) Additional elements of informed consent. When appropriate, one or more of the following elements of information shall also be provided to each subject:

(1) A statement that the particular treatment or procedure may involve risks to the subject (or to the embryo or fetus, if the subject is or may become pregnant), which are currently unforeseeable;

(2) Anticipated circumstances under which the subject's participation may be terminated by the investigator without regard to the subject's consent;

(3) Any additional costs to the subject that may result from participation in the research;

(4) The consequences of a subject's decision to withdraw from the research and procedures for orderly termination of participation by the subject;

(5) A statement that significant new findings developed during the course of the research, which may relate to the subject's willingness to continue participation will be provided to the subject; and

(6) The approximate number of subjects involved in the study.

REQUIRED ELEMENTS

Required Element 1—The Research Declaration

The consent document must include a declaration that the project involves research. As medical research often involves treatments, and these treatments may include consents for standard interventions (such as a procedure or test), the inclusion of this component should be positioned at the beginning of the document to ensure that the potential research subject is aware from the outset that the subsequent discussion is focused on research.

Required Element 2—Identification of Foreseeable Risks or Discomforts

The researcher is obligated to inform the research subjects about known risks and discomforts or added burdens (such as time commitments) that may occur as a result of participation in the research study. Although all known risks must be included, it is general practice to indicate the expected severity and anticipated frequency at which the known risks may occur. This is most easily accomplished by including a table that identifies risks and assigns an approximation of frequency and severity to each.

Required Element 3—Identification of Possible Benefits

In many instances, the research participant will not benefit directly from taking part in the study. In such cases, the potential benefit that may accrue to science and society should be outlined. If there are potential benefits to participants, they should be identified clearly. Remuneration for participation is not considered a benefit of participation and should not be included in this section.

Required Element 4—Alternatives to Participation

Any person who is being asked to consent to participate in a research protocol must be informed about any alternative(s) that may exist. In some instances, there may be no viable alternative to the intervention that is being studied in the research protocol. In such instances, the contrast is clear and the participation by a potential subject is not likely to be influenced by the existence of ineffective or poorly effective alternatives. In other cases, there may well be established and approved alternatives to the intervention under study, and the investigator is obligated to present these as viable options. It also is important to convey to the potential subject that, by participating in the research study, s/he may forego other approved therapies. For this reason, the investigator must clearly explain to the subject what alternatives exist and the implications of participating in the study.

Required Element 5—Confidentiality

Disclosure of the extent to which confidentiality of personal and medical information will be protected is another required component of the informed consent document. This section of the consent document should specify how the medical and personal information is going to be collected, how it will be used, and what measures will be taken to keep it secure. The specific language used by many IRBs to satisfy this element has been influenced substantially by the Health Insurance Portability and Accountability Act of 1996 (HIPAA). The HIPAA Privacy Rule requires that research subjects specifically authorize use and/or disclosure of their protected health information (PHI). This can be accomplished in the research-informed consent document or in a separate authorization form.

Required Element 6—Compensation

Specific mention must be made of any compensation that the participant will receive in exchange for their participation. In addition to detailing what compensation the subject may receive—if any—it is important to identify what study-related expenses will be covered and/or reimbursed. This can be challenging when a research includes procedures or tests that are considered "standard of care," and for which the subject or insurer may be responsible. As with an assessment of medical risks of participation, such information permits a clear assessment of the financial risks that can accompany participation in a study.

Required Element 7—Contact Information

Contact information must be listed for the investigators. This provides the research subject the ability to contact a member of the research team if s/he should have questions or if problems should arise. Contact information should be provided that allows accessibility to the researchers both during and outside of office hours.

Required Element 8—Participation Is Voluntary

This item may seem self-explanatory but is required to establish with certainty that the potential research subject understands that his/her participation in the project is completely voluntary and that a decision to decline will not result in punishment or any loss of privileges to which they otherwise would be entitled.

ADDITIONAL ELEMENTS

In addition to the required elements described above, there are six additional components that are identified in 45 CFR § 46.111 as elements that should be provided when appropriate **(Table 3-4)**. These elements either address specific circumstances (e.g., risks to the fetus) or provide additional details regarding the size of the study, the rules under which the study is to be conducted, or the financial implications of participating in the study. These elements are treated as required components of informed consent documents by many institutional review boards. A template that incorporates all of these elements can be found in Appendix A.

GUIDELINES FOR PREPARING CONSENT FORMS AND ASSURING AN EFFECTIVE AND VALID CONSENTING PROCESS

Informed consent documents attempt to convey a large amount of information in a single document. Careful attention to the phrasing of the document can have a profound effect on how easily the information may be understood. Word choice, sentence length and structure, and education level of the vocabulary are particularly important in creating text that is comprehensive, yet easy to understand. A list of several helpful tips to keep in mind while writing the consent document is provided in **Table 3-5**.

The creation of an understandable consent document is challenging, but is only one element in the consenting process. The consent document serves to document the

TABLE **3-5** | Tips to Remember When Writing Informed Consent Documents

General Considerations
• Use simple, common words (avoid medical terminology or jargon)
• Always use "you" to address the reader
• Explain and define technical terms
• Avoid if possible long words with many syllables and unnecessary adjectives
• Avoid legal jargon
• Avoid abbreviations and acronyms
• Try to use the same words consistently

Sentence Structure and Paragraphs
• Keep sentences short (8 to 10 words is good)
• Use a conversational tone
• Avoid complex sentence structures
• Consider breaking into a short list when there are more than 3 points to the sentence
• Avoid long paragraphs
• Keep one idea per paragraph
• Utilize list and bullet points when possible
• Keep sections short
• Use visuals like pictures or diagrams when appropriate

Formatting
• Standardize the layout throughout the document.

TABLE **3-6** | Barriers to an Effective Informed Consent Process

• Using highly technical language
• Rushing through the explanation of the procedures and risks
• Not pausing to allow the subject to ask questions
• Inability to detect subject's lack of understanding and comprehension of the general purpose of the research and the potential risks
• Not showing appropriate concern for problems voiced by subject
• Subject's lack of understanding their right to withdraw at anytime
• Subject's lack of understanding that withdrawal will not influence other treatment options
• Subject's lack of understanding of the differences between traditional, individualized clinical care and standardized treatment during research participation

conversation between the potential subject and the investigator. The process of informed consent begins with recruitment materials and continues throughout the life of the study. Permitting sufficient time for explanation and discussion relating to the study and its objectives, procedures, and risks is critical. **Table 3-6** outlines several common barriers that can detract from the process of obtaining valid informed consent.

DOCUMENTATION OF INFORMED CONSENT

The Federal regulations and Good Clinical Practice guidance (GCP) require that informed consent be documented. This is typically done by giving a copy of the signed informed consent form to the subject, and keeping a copy with the study records. However, GCP guidelines go further. In order to satisfy GCP requirements, one must also document that

- the subject has had ample time and opportunity to ask questions, and
- the version of the informed consent form that was signed by the subject is approved by the IRB.

An easy way to do this is by using a checklist when obtaining consent. Appendix B provides a sample checklist. It also is a good idea to document the subjects' understanding of the research project before obtaining consent. Note, documentation of a subject's understanding of the research project is not a federal regulation or GCP requirement; however, it is good practice. One way of accomplishing this is by having the subject complete a worksheet demonstrating knowledge and understanding of the research project. Appendix C provides a sample worksheet.

WHAT ACTIVITIES ARE SUBJECT TO IRB REVIEW?

Not all research activities will require IRB review. In general, any activity that meets either the Department of Health and Human Services (DHHS) definition of both "research" and "human subjects" or the Food and Drug Administration (FDA) definitions of both "clinical investigation" and "human subjects" is considered human research and requires review and approval by an IRB.

Research means a systematic investigation, including research development, testing and evaluation, designed to develop or contribute to generalizable knowledge (45 CFR § 46.102[d]).

"Human subject" means a living individual about whom an investigator (whether professional or student) conducting research obtains (1) data through intervention or interaction with the individual or (2) identifiable private information (45 CFR § 46.102[f]).

The comparable FDA regulation (21 CFR 50) does not define "research" per se; rather, it defines "clinical investigation" as "any experiment that involves a test article and one or more human subjects …" (21 CFR § 50.3[c]).

The following are examples of activities that generally are not considered "human subject research" and do not require IRB approval:

- **Deidentified Commercially Available Human Cells or Cell Lines:** IRB review is not required since deidentified human cells or cell lines acquired from established vendors and government tissue banks do not meet the regulatory definition of human subject research. When human cells are obtained from one of these repositories, investigators are reminded to review the contract or purchase agreement carefully to ensure that the planned use of the specimens will be in accordance with the vendor's or supplier's terms and conditions.

- **Specimens from an IRB-Approved Tissue Repository:** IRB review is not required if (1) the specimens are deidentified or (2) the specimens are coded, but the investigator will not be provided the link or other identifiers under any circumstances.

- **Fee-for-Service Analysis of Human Specimens:** IRB review is not required for activities limited to the performance of analyses on human specimens as a commercial or genuinely noncollaborative service. For example, appropriately qualified laboratory staff may perform analyses of blood samples for investigators solely on a commercial (noncollaborative) basis. In such situations, the personnel performing the analyses are not considered to be "engaged in the research," but still must adhere to the commonly recognized professional standards for maintaining privacy and confidentiality.

- **Public Health Surveillance:** IRB review generally is not required for activities that are ongoing as a part of routine medical and public health care functions for preventing and controlling disease or injury (may include emergent or urgently identified or suspected imminent health threats to the population to document the existence and magnitude).

- **Quality Improvement and Quality Assurance:** IRB review is not required for many types of quality improvement and quality assurance activities. Only those QI and QA projects that also meet the federal definition of human research require IRB review.

- **Case Reports:** IRB review is not required for presenting medical information collected from a clinical activity rather than a research activity. Case reports describe a unique treatment, case, or outcome. The examination of the case is not systematic, and there is usually no data analysis or testing of a hypothesis. Investigators must ensure that the HIPAA privacy rules are followed with respect to using or accessing PHI (a HIPAA Authorization may be required).

- **Cadaver Tissue:** Federal regulations do not require IRB review for use of cadaveric tissue or decedent data because the regulations cover only living humans and private information about living humans. However, some states have passed laws requiring IRB review for research on cadavers and decedent data so it is important to be familiar with your state's laws.

WAIVERS AND ALTERATIONS OF INFORMED CONSENT

Informed consent is a critical tool for protection of human research subjects. Unless an IRB approves a waiver of informed consent or a waiver of the documentation of informed consent (i.e., verbal consent), investigators are responsible for obtaining and documenting informed consent from each research subject or from their legally authorized representatives.

IRBs have the latitude to grant consent waivers and to permit verbal consent. In addition, an IRB may approve a consent procedure that does not include, or which alters, some or all of the elements of informed consent. To approve an altered consent or a waiver of consent, an IRB must find and document that

1. The research or demonstration project is to be conducted by or subject to the approval of state or local government officials and is designed to study, evaluate, or otherwise examine:
   (i) public benefit or service programs;
   (ii) procedures for obtaining benefits or services under those programs;
   (iii) possible changes in or alternatives to those programs or procedures; or
   (iv) possible changes in methods or levels of payment for benefits or services under those programs
2. And the research could not practicably be carried out without the waiver or alteration.

Or

1. The research involves no more than minimal risk to the subjects;
2. The waiver or alteration will not adversely affect the rights and welfare of the subjects;
3. The research could not practicably be carried out without the waiver or alteration; and
4. Whenever appropriate, the subjects will be provided with additional pertinent information after participation.

When an IRB waives the requirement to obtain informed consent, it waives the entire requirement for informed consent process. However, when the IRB grants an alteration of some or all of the elements of the informed consent (e.g., removes a required element of consent from the document), the process of obtaining informed consent is still required. Scenarios that might be exempt from all or some of the informed consent requirements are shown in **Table 3-7**.

TABLE **3-7** | **Examples of Waivers or Alterations of Informed Consent Elements**

Waiver of written documentation of informed consent

With this waiver, the investigator would be required to read or provide the informed consent form to a subject, but would not need to obtain the subject's signature on the consent form. Examples of when this waiver might be applicable would be some internet or phone surveys or when signing the form might have some negative consequence for the subject. It must be emphasized that these waivers will be given only when there are compelling reasons for doing so.

Waiver or alteration of informed consent

With this waiver, the investigator may provide to the subject a consent that does not include or alter one or all of the required elements. Examples of when this waiver might be applicable would be when a researcher is conducting secondary data analysis and the subjects cannot be located or when requiring informed consent might somehow actually have negative consequences for research subjects.

WAIVER OF DOCUMENTATION OF INFORMED CONSENT (VERBAL CONSENT)

In some instances, verbal consent without a written form may be appropriate. The regulations at 45 CFR § 46.117 allow the IRB to waive the requirement for the investigator to obtain a signed consent form for some or all subjects if it finds either:

- The only record linking the subject and the research project would be the consent document;
- The principal risk would be potential harm resulting from a breach of confidentiality;
- Each participant will be asked whether the participant wants documentation linking the participant with the research, and the participant's wishes will govern; and
- The research is not a clinical investigation subject to FDA regulations.

Or

- The research presents no more than minimal risk of harm to participants and
- The research involves no procedures for which written consent is normally required outside of the research context.

In cases where the documentation requirement for informed consent is waived, an IRB can require the researchers to provide participants with a written statement or information sheet regarding the research. This written statement or information sheet requires IRB approval.

Researchers interested in obtaining a waiver of written (signed) informed consent should make sure that their research meets the criteria listed above.

NON-ENGLISH-SPEAKING SUBJECTS AND TRANSLATION OF CONSENT DOCUMENTS

To ensure that the burdens and benefits of research are fairly distributed, federal regulations (45 CFR § 46.111) for the protection of human research subjects require that IRBs consider whether selection of subjects is equitable. A related ethical principle is that the target sample for a study should be representative of the population that has the potential to benefit from participation in the research. For this reason, IRBs may require the inclusion of non-English-speaking persons in research unless there is a compelling justification for their exclusion.

Examples of acceptable justifications include but are not limited to:

1. Study requires use of data collection instruments, such as survey instruments, that have not been validated scientifically in languages other than English;
2. Study will include participants already known to the principal investigator and who all speak English (this often is the case for "follow-up" studies in which only a known group of current subjects will be eligible to participate in the second phase of study);
3. Study is of a disease or disorder so rare that local enrollment is expected to be five or less; or

4. Study involves significant risk or complexity related to the condition under study, the test article, or both that requires ability to efficiently communicate throughout the study execution in the situation where study personnel may not be able to speak languages other than English and resources for translation services are not available.

Federal regulations (45 CFR § 46.116 and § 46.117) also require that informed consent information be presented "in language understandable to the subject" and, in most situations, that informed consent be documented in writing. Where informed consent is documented in accordance with § 46.117(b)(1), the written consent document should embody, in language understandable to the subject, all the elements necessary for legally effective informed consent.

When a potential research subject expresses interest in participating in a study and is unable to speak or read English, they must be presented with a translated informed consent document, unless the IRB has approved the use of a so-called "short form" that summarizes all the required elements of informed consent for research used in conjunction with the content of the full consent form discussed with the potential subject in their primary language. Investigators should plan ahead for expected subject populations who are unable to speak or read English and should arrange for translation of the IRB-approved English informed consent/assent form prior to beginning study recruitment. The informed consent process is the same as for English-speaking subjects; however, in many institutions, a qualified interpreter must be present to facilitate the consent conversation between the investigator and the potential subject prior to enrollment. This requirement is not uniformly enforced at all institutions.

When non-English speakers will be enrolled, a professional translation of the complete consent/assent form(s) is required unless the IRB has granted a waiver of documentation of informed consent or has approved the use of an abbreviated consent form (short form). Translated forms must be approved by the IRB prior to use.

DNA AND UNUSED SAMPLES

An increasing focus of human research is the interplay between genetics and human disease. For this reason, an increasing number of investigations include the use of samples to study genetic or other biologic attributes and relate them to the subject matter of the investigations. Whether the material maintains linkage to the patient's identity or deidentified, it is important that the use(s) of such material be fully disclosed and adequately described within the informed consent document. In many instances, this disclosure and consent is contained within the overall consent document; in other instances, a separate consent form may be required (Appendix D) (see Chapter 4).

HIPAA AUTHORIZATION AND WAIVER OF AUTHORIZATIONS

HIPAA is an acronym for the Health Insurance Portability and Accountability Act of 1996 (http://www.hhs.gov/ocr/privacy/). While the primary purpose of HIPAA was to enable employees and their families to transfer health care benefits from one employer to another, or to continue coverage in the case of a job loss, the aspects of the law that deal specifically with data security and privacy are commonly referred to as The Privacy Rule.

The Privacy Rule establishes a minimum standard for the protection of protected health information (PHI), which is defined as individually identifiable health information that is transmitted or maintained in any medium. Human research subject protection regulations include some provisions that are similar to, but distinct from, the Privacy Rule's provisions for creation, use, and dissemination of research data. The Privacy Rule expanded privacy protections, which apply regardless of the study-funding source.

The Privacy Rule recognizes the need for researchers to access, use, and disclose PHI for a wide range of research activities, and provides various ways in which researchers can access and use the information necessary for research. Of particular importance is The Privacy Rule's requirement that written authorization (HIPAA Authorization) be obtained from the subject for the use of PHI for research purposes (unless an exception applies).

For research activities involving PHI, some IRB's will act as the institution's Privacy Board (required by HIPAA) to review and approve the proposed access, use, and disclosure of the PHI. The Privacy Board/IRB is responsible for determining whether research subjects are required to sign an authorization (HIPAA Authorization) for the use and disclosure of their PHI, or if one of the exceptions to the authorization requirements may apply. Examples of these exceptions include waivers of authorization and the use of deidentified data or limited data sets.

It is important to note that although the laws govern the use of PHI for research, these regulations are implemented differently by different IRBs. At some institutions, the elements required for the HIPAA authorization are contained within the study informed consent document itself. At other institutions, the elements are contained in a separate document (HIPAA Authorization). For this reason, in this chapter, both are discussed separately and separate templates are provided. A template of a HIPAA authorization is contained in Appendix E. An informed consent template containing both elements is provided in Appendix F.

It is important for researchers to become familiar with how and under what conditions PHI can be accessed, used, and disclosed for research purposes.

HIPAA WAIVER OF AUTHORIZATION

As stated above, in most situations the regulations require that a signed HIPAA authorization be obtained before the PHI of a subject can be acquired, used or disclosed for research purposes. A waiver of this authorization requirement allows an investigator to acquire, use, or disclose health information without securing such an authorization.

The IRB/Privacy Board may grant a waiver of the authorization requirement if several regulatory criteria can be fulfilled. One criterion is key: the research could not *practicably* be conducted without the waiver. If it will be difficult or impossible to obtain a signed authorization from the potential research subjects, the study may qualify for a waiver of authorization.

Situations in which the request for a waiver of authorization may be appropriate include:

- research on existing health information, that is, medical records research and
- research where a waiver of informed consent also is being requested, that is, survey research via phone.

The four criteria that must be satisfied for a *full* waiver of authorization are:

1. The research could not practicably be conducted without the waiver or alteration of authorization, that is, there is no other mechanism available that would permit you to obtain the information needed for study recruitment under HIPAA.
2. The research could not practicably be conducted without access to and use of the health information sought in the waiver.
3. A brief description of the health information for which use or access has been determined to be necessary. The waiver will permit the researcher to access only this information.
4. The use or disclosure of health information involves no more than a minimal risk to the privacy of individuals, based on, at least, the presence of the following elements:
   • An adequate plan to protect the identifiers from improper use and disclosure;
   • An adequate plan to destroy the identifiers at the earliest opportunity consistent with conduct of the research, unless there is a health or research justification for retaining the identifiers or such retention is otherwise required by law; and
   • Adequate written assurances are provided that the PHI will not be reused or disclosed to any other person or entity, except as required by law, for authorized oversight of the research study, or for other research for which the use or disclosure of PHI would be permitted.

A template containing the required elements of a HIPAA Waiver of Authorization can be found in Appendix G.

A *partial waiver*, or *alteration*, of the HIPAA authorization may also be granted by the IRB/Privacy Board in cases where granting a full waiver of authorization is not warranted. These additional mechanisms allow the IRB to alter or eliminate one or more of the regulatory elements normally required in the HIPAA authorization. Investigators should consult with their institutional IRB for more information on these options.

THE PROCESS OF OBTAINING INFORMED CONSENT

The consent process is more than what is contained within the consent document itself. The act of obtaining informed consent is an educational process that involves explanation, the opportunity to ask questions regarding benefits and risks, and deliberation about the choices presented. Viewed from this perspective, the informed consent document is simply a guide to the elements that must be covered during the consent conversation(s) and a form of documentation that consent was obtained. The entirety of this process is critical to ensure that participants are fully informed as to the benefits and risks of the research and attendant procedures and have consented voluntarily based on this information.

CHAPTER 4

Ethics of Data Sharing and Handling of Genetic Information

Bradley A. Malin, PhD, David Karp, MD, PhD, and Richard H. Scheuermann, PhD

INTRODUCTION

A number of organizations, distributed around the globe, have invested considerable effort to construct information technology infrastructure to support the management and analysis of data on human participants enrolled in clinical and translational research studies (1). Organizations are now moving toward models of broader data sharing and accessibility through open-access translational research information systems (OTRIS). OTRIS are dynamic and evolving, in terms of technical implementation and oversight, but have a common goal of establishing data warehousing infrastructure to facilitate the rapid dissemination of research findings. They aim to integrate a variety of data types, such as experimental information derived from laboratory experimentation (e.g., genome sequence, gene expression, and proteomics data) with rich clinical phenotypes. OTRIS further aim to integrate data from various laboratories and other resources, so that the research community has access to a broad range of datasets to validate and reanalyze published findings, as well

41

as mine for novel clinically relevant discoveries. Thus, it is the intention of OTRIS managers to make their systems and, to the extent to which it is possible, the data within freely accessible as a resource to the public.

OTRIS raise complex ethical, legal, and social issues that developers, managers, and scientists associated with these systems will need to consider as software engineering and scientific investigation moves forward (1–3). Recent meetings have solicited information from ethicists, informaticists, lawyers, and biomedical scientists to characterize various issues associated with the construction of database archives, ranging from informed consent to attribution of property to identifiability of human participants in supported research projects (4). In this chapter, we elaborate on the data privacy issues in the context of OTRIS. We recognize that a complete solution will require further investigation on ethical, social, and legal components of the problem, but we use this forum to illustrate how policy and technology can be combined to resolve data sharing and privacy goals.

It has been stressed that the availability of OTRIS for widespread use is contingent on the protection of patient anonymity (5). And, while biomedical privacy policies and technologies exist, various studies suggest they are ill-equipped for environments that centralize detailed patient-specific data (6). Moreover, recent forensic science research (7,8) has prompted significant changes to data sharing policies for various OTRIS, most notably the database of Genotype and Phenotype (dbGaP) (9) at the U.S. National Library of Medicine (10). In the face of such threats, one must question if there are potential privacy vulnerabilities for other emerging resources. Furthermore, if such threats do exist, then what are the measures, both from a technical and policy perspective, that should be explored to mitigate such threats?

In this chapter, we illustrate how OTRIS are vulnerable, but it is important to note that not all emerging OTRIS are susceptible to privacy violations in the same manner. In addition, the power that responsible policies and oversight can provide in mitigating threats that remain in deidentified research settings should not be neglected. The issues raised and potential solutions offered in this chapter are applicable to many informatics resources intending to share clinical and biological data for translational research purposes, and where possible, we draw on examples from emerging OTRIS to demonstrate their potential application.

POLICIES AND REQUIREMENTS

Before we address technical issues, it is important to note the regulatory landscape. Data collected, shared, and used within OTRIS will be subject to various regulatory controls. The appropriateness of such controls depends on from where the data will be derived. In particular, there are several primary privacy and data sharing policies that OTRIS managers must be cognizant of as they move forward. The following is an introduction to some of the relevant regulatory issues at play and should not be considered a comprehensive list.

NIH Data Sharing Policy

The National Institutes of Health (NIH) Data Sharing Policy was designed to increase access to data collected through, or studied with, federal funding (11). The policy applies to all projects that receive at least $500,000 in annual direct funding. According to the policy, data must be shared in a "deidentified" format in a manner similar to the Safe Harbor model as defined in the Privacy Rule of the Health Insurance Portability and Accountability Act (see below). The data sharer must also remove information for which there is prior knowledge that the information could be used to determine the identity of the subjects. Some investigators have argued that the sensitivity of their datasets and the lack of ability to provide provable privacy guarantees are sufficient to opt out of data sharing.

NIH GWAS Policy

Genome-wide genetic scans of sequence variations have become important, but costly, research tools for the biomedical community. The NIH created a specific policy for the collection and sharing of data derived from, or studied in, genome-wide association studies (GWAS)(12). Similar to the 2003 data sharing policy, the GWAS policy was defined such that it applies to any project regardless of funding level in which genome-wide genetic scans are produced or studied. The NIH has since designated dbGaP as the repository to which NIH-sponsored investigators should submit their GWAS records. As in the NIH Data Sharing Policy, GWAS data must be deidentified prior to dissemination.

The NIH has recognized that genomic data itself may lead to the reidentification of an individual. Thus, users of GWAS datasets in dbGaP must sign a contractual use agreement that explicitly prohibits nonsanctioned uses, as well as attempts to identify subjects (see below). Other NIH groups and repositories are applying similar use agreements to assign legal constraints to the use of information stored in their OTRIS.

HIPAA Privacy Rule and Data Sharing

In the United States, when a "covered entity," as defined by HIPAA (e.g., health care providers and health data clearinghouses), wishes to share the data collected in the context of clinical activities, it must adhere to the Privacy Rule (13) (see Chapter 2). The regulation outlines several routes by which personal health information can be shared without patient consent for secondary research purposes: (1) Safe Harbor, (2) Limited Data Set, and (3) Statistical Certification.

The *Safe Harbor Standard* allows covered entities to publicly share data once they are stripped of an enumerated list of 18 types of personal identifiers. These include explicit identifiers (e.g., names), "quasi-identifiers" (e.g., dates and geocodes), and traceable elements (e.g., medical record numbers). Neither clinical nor genomic data are explicitly labeled as a personal identifier, and it has been debated if such data can be released under this policy (14). For years, clinical data have been shared in public resources, such as hospital discharge databases (15,16). Similarly, person-specific DNA sequences have been disclosed to public repositories, such as those at the National Center for Biotechnology Information (NCBI) (17).

Various groups argue against disclosing data via Safe Harbor based on the observations that the usefulness of such data for certain types of studies (e.g., epidemiology) is questionable, but also out of "reidentification" concerns (5,18). Rather, an alternative called the *Limited Data Set Standard* is advocated, which allows covered entities to share more detailed data, including dates and zip codes. The tradeoff is that data recipients must enter into an acceptable use contract that prohibits reidentification. While this policy is appropriate for trusted investigators, as the quantity of centralized data and number of investigators granted access increases, such an approach may become infeasible to manage. Moreover, this policy neither prevents an individual from attempting reidentification nor assesses the risk of reidentification.

The *Statistical Standard* allows sharing data in any format, provided an expert certifies "the risk is very small that the information could be used by the recipient, alone or in combination with other reasonably available information, to identify an individual" (13). Methods to quantify risks have been researched (7,18), but no standards have emerged. One disclosure control method that has been considered is to "perturb" DNA sequences, for example, AACCTATA shared as AATCAATA (19). The intuition is that as the quantity of perturbation increases, the likelihood that an investigator can determine the original sequence decreases, implying greater privacy protection. The tradeoff, however, is that perturbation can potentially obscure, or worse, lead to false, associations. Thus, it could diminish the utility and scientific credibility of the resource. A second criticism of such a protection approach is that research has shown that certain types of perturbation can be filtered to reliably infer the original data (20). Despite such problems, data protection based on scientific models can be achieved, but care must be taken to design them with formal principles.

REIDENTIFICATION MODELS, METHODS, AND APPLICATIONS

As we alluded to, data that are deidentified according to the aforementioned polices can be "reidentified" to the individuals from which the data were derived via numerous routes. As we illustrate in **Figure 4-1**, reidentification is a process and requires the satisfaction of certain conditions. First, it requires that the deidentified data are unique or "distinguishing." In other words, we must be able to pinpoint an individual in a group of size *n* people or less. Genomic sequence data, for instance, and possibly other laboratory and molecular expression data are often highly distinguishing. However, it needs to be recognized that the ability to distinguish data is, by itself, insufficient to claim that the corresponding individual's privacy will actually be compromised. This is because of the second condition, which is that we need a "naming" resource. Without such a resource, there is no way to link the

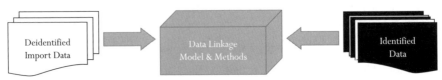

FIGURE **4-1**   A general model of data "reidentification." There are three conditions that need to be satisfied: the ability to distinguish an individual's record in *(1)* deidentified and *(2)* identified resources, and *(3)* a mechanism for relating (or linking) data from the resources.

deidentified data to an identity.[1] Finally, for the third condition, we need a mechanism to relate the deidentified and identified resources. Inability to design such a relational mechanism would hamper an adversary's opportunity to achieve success to no better than random assignment of deidentified data and named individuals.

There are many situations in which deidentified biomedical information can be reidentified to the patient from whom it was derived without hacking or breaking into private health information systems. For instance, in the mid-1990s it was shown that deidentified hospital discharge records, which were publicly available at the state level, could be linked to identified public records in the form of voter registration lists. The result received notoriety because it led to the reidentification of the medical status of the governor of the Commonwealth of Massachusetts (21). This attack was achieved by linking the resources on the seemingly innocuous, but common, fields of patient's date of birth, gender, and zip code. Various estimates indicate that the uniqueness of this combination of attributes in the U.S. population is somewhere between 65% and 87%, and with certain subpopulations even more unique (22,23).

Risk of Identification

One of the responses to the aforementioned attack was the HIPAA Safe Harbor policy. But, it should be recognized that even the suppression of all enumerated features fails to prevent *all* reidentifications. In many instances, there are residual features, including the remaining demographics (e.g., race, year of birth, state of residence, and gender) that can lead to identification. However, the extent to which residual features can be applied to reidentification is context-dependent and relies on the availability of the fields that can be leveraged in the attack. In **Table 4-1**, we provide some general guidelines to consider

TABLE **4-1** | A Summary of OTRIS Data Reidentification Assessment Mechanisms

Replication	Prioritize OTRIS data attributes into different levels of risk, according to their replicability (e.g., molecular expression data are less replicable than genomic sequence data)
Resources	Determine which external resources contain the subject's identities as well as the replicable attributes in the OTRIS data
Distinguish	Determine the extent to which subject's deidentified data can be distinguished in the OTRIS (e.g., it is easier to distinguish an individual using 100 SNPs as opposed to 1 SNP)
Access	Determine who has access to the identified resources? Is the data publicly available? Is it a more private resource?
Assess risk	The greater the replicability, the availability, and distinguishability of OTRIS data, the greater the risk for reidentification (and vice versa)

---

[1]We recognize that the lack of a readily available naming resource does not imply that data are sufficiently protected from reidentification. Nonetheless, it does indicate that it is much harder to identify an individual, or group of individuals, given the resources at hand.

when assessing the reidentification risk of data in OTRIS. In general, it helps to partition the person-specific features into classes of relatively "high" and relatively "low" risk. We recognize that risk is more of a continuous variable, but this type of dichotomization helps illustrate how context impacts risk. Beyond riskiness of attributes, it is important to understand the routes by which data can be linked to naming sources or sensitive knowledge can be inferred, as we review below.

High-Risk Identifiers

Higher risk features are those that are documented in multiple environments and are publicly available. These are features that can be exploited by any recipient of such records. For instance, patient or research subject demographics are high-risk identifiers. Even the demographics that are permissive under the Safe Harbor policy leave certain individuals in a unique status and thus at nontrivial risk for identification through public resources that contain similar features, such as birth, death, marriage, voter, property assessor records, and more.

Low-Risk Identifiers

Lower risk features are those that do not appear in public records and are less readily available. For instance, clinical features, such as an individual's diagnoses and treatments, are relatively static (i.e., because they are often mapped to standard coding terminologies for billing purposes) and can manifest in deidentified resources, such as the aforementioned hospital discharge databases as well as identified resources, such as electronic medical records. While combinations of diagnosis and treatment codes, or temporal dependencies, can uniquely characterize a patient in a population (24), the identified records are available to a much smaller group of individuals than the general public. Moreover, this select group of individuals may be relatively more trustworthy, such as care providers and business associates of the organization that generated the documented features. Additional disincentives may exist as well, such as HIPAA-related penalties that are applied in the event an individual willingly violates the terms of employment to commit a breach of privacy.

Biosample Data

When OTRIS include data derived from biological samples, the situation becomes a bit more complex. In certain instances the information that is associated with genomic and expression data, particularly genomic data derived from a clinical setting, permits relationships to be established between deidentified and identifiable resources. The following is a summary of several attacks, with further details available elsewhere (6).

Genotype–Phenotype

There exists an inherent relationship between certain genomic data sequences and physical phenotypic manifestations. A clinical phenotype may be described in biomedical coding standards, such as the International Classification of Diseases (ICD), and may be disclosed in various settings, including "semiprivate" data, such as administrative or insurance records, but also more public records, such as hospital discharge databases.

Familial Information

A second type of attack is made possible because genomic data is increasingly disseminated in the context of familial information. This practice is common in gene-hunting expeditions. Familial information could be represented in the format of a deidentified pedigree, which reports gender, disease status, and the death status of the family members. At the same time, there are a variety of publicly available identified information available. One particular resource that has been exploited for identifiers is obituaries, which have wide coverage on a population and are often free to post in newspapers. Such resources tend to include information on the recently deceased individual as well as the family relations (25).

Trails and Location-Based Patterns

Many patients (and research participants) are transient and visit multiple institutions providing care. As such, a patient's location–visit pattern is often distinguishing and facilitates what has been termed a "trails" attack (26). In this scenario, a patient visits multiple hospitals, where his clinical and DNA-related data are collected. The facilities forward deidentified DNA records, tagged with the submitting institution, to a public centralized databank (27–29). Additionally, the hospitals send identifiable discharge records, including patient demographics and diagnoses to a discharge database (30). Even if there is no clear biomedical relationship between the diagnosis codes and sequence markers in the DNA, we can track the hospitals a patient has visited (i.e., the "trail") in the discharge data and the DNA records in the repository (26). Notably, this attack is generalizable in that trails can manifest in a number of environments (31).

Genome Sequence Data

Genome sequence data are increasingly applied in clinical research. However, it is also a well-known distinguishing feature unto itself. Lin and colleagues (19) demonstrated that only a small number ($<$ 100) of single-nucleotide polymorphisms, or SNPs, is required to uniquely characterize an individual in the entire world's population. SNP data are increasingly found in ancestry, clinical, molecular phenotype, and pharmaceutical efficacy association studies. Thus, if an adversary has access to an identified DNA sequence, it may be possible to learn additional information about the individual from the deidentified data in the association studies.

In recognition of this fact, dbGaP decided to publicly disseminate SNP–clinical status correlations for various datasets only as aggregated results. Specifically, for each dataset and for each individual SNP, it publicly posted the proportion of the population that was diagnosed with (or without) a clinical feature (e.g., immunodeficiency disorder) and the corresponding SNP value.

However, as was recently demonstrated by Homer and colleagues (7,8), such an approach does not prevent privacy threats. They demonstrated what we call a "pool attack," where the information on several thousand SNPs could be used to determine if an identified individual's DNA was in the set of clinically positive cases, the set of clinically negative cases, or neither of the above. Moreover, the approach involved in the attack is *applicable* to any environment in which aggregate statistics on biomedical datasets is available. Details of their attack are beyond the scope of this chapter, but can be found elsewhere. This attack is important to note because it had significant impact on dbGaP's public data access policy (as described in the Observations section).

Laboratory Reports and Expression Data

The previous types of data and attacks may compromise privacy because they are sufficiently replicable and available in multiple datasets. However, data stored in many OTRIS are also expected to consist of functional genomics data (e.g., gene expression microarray data) derived from laboratory testing. While such data may be unique and located in multiple datasets, the extent to which these data are replicable is questionable. To the best of our knowledge there is limited research that addresses the precision of repeated functional genomics tests. However, if such information is not adequately replicable, these data may be considered less risky to share than sequence data.

OBSERVATIONS

Before proposing specific recommendations regarding technologies and policies to improve data privacy protections, we wish to return to the pool attack and highlight several results and policy decisions. The pool attack did not involve a compromise of identity because the adversary was already in possession of the subject's identity and genomic data. However, the attack resulted in a breach of confidentiality because the subject did not inform the adversary of their clinical status. Given the accuracy of the attack, the NIH felt they could not publish statistical summaries of SNP–clinical class correlations without violating the privacy principles stated in their data sharing policies. As a consequence, the NIH removed all summary statistics from the public version of dbGaP (10). Following the lead of the NIH, the Wellcome Trust, the main biobanking and human genomic data dissemination agency in the United Kingdom, followed suit. The policy changes received significant attention from the popular media (32–35). While privacy advocates have lauded these actions, there are several reasons why this response is not necessarily appropriate for every OTRIS.

Observation 1: The attack requires an identified reference sample. The attack is a feasible attack in that it can be achieved given relatively open data sharing strategies. In fact, the approach is generalizable to other types of information derived from biological samples. However, the question remains as to what the likelihood of such an attack is given today's climate. To achieve the attack, the adversary needs access to an identified DNA sequence, which begs the question of who would be in possession of such information? It has been suggested that such information could be available through forensic investigations, but it is unclear if forensic specialists would be sufficiently motivated to learn clinical information about the subject in question. Second, it has been noted that individuals beyond the forensic realm could collect biological samples, subsequently sequence, and use the resulting information, but the economic and computational barriers are nontrivial and it is not clear that anyone would attempt to mount such an attack. This is not to say that such an attack could not be committed by motivated individuals, but that the context for executing such an attack has yet to be clearly voiced. We recognize that biological data will be increasingly available as high-throughput genomic sequencing technology becomes cheaper and more mainstream, but at the present time, the threat is believed to be more theoretical than practical.

Observation 2: Regulating aggregate results and microdata in the same manner is a potentially restrictive administrative model. Investigators conducting NIH-sponsored GWAS are encouraged to submit their deidentified records to dbGaP (12). The result is that dbGaP stores datasets for a number of NIH institutes. Initially, dbGaP defined its access policy according to a two-tier model. The first tier consisted of "public" information, which included summary information for each dataset, including data collection mechanisms, the types of demographic, clinical, and biological information collected, and summary statistics for the various "classes" of individuals. This was designated as public information that was readily available on the dbGaP website. The second tier of access was for person-level records or "microdata." To access this information, investigators must proceed through a formal evaluation process. The process begins when a new investigator submits a request to access the records in a dataset. The application is sent to an NIH data access committee (DAC). Since each dataset may have unique use limitations and may have been sponsored by a different NIH institute, the investigator may need to make multiple requests for multiple datasets.

When the NIH decided that summary statistics for data deposited in dbGaP would no longer be accessible through the first, or public, access level, such information was moved to the second tier. However, the DAC model was designed to handle requests for individual-level datasets to validate or explore specific hypotheses, not requests to mine for new knowledge *across* datasets that are unrelated in the initial reasons for their collection. Thus, this approach to managing summary information could limit large-scale data mining and hypothesis-generation-driven research methodologies that are gaining popularity in the biomedical domain.

Observation 3: Technical and statistical measures can be applied to disseminate person-specific GWAS data with privacy risk guarantees. From a technical perspective, the removal of summary statistics from the public realm created an "all or nothing" data access setting. Initially, researchers were permitted access to "all" of the SNPs and the relative occurrence of variant statistics, but after the policy change, researchers were shuttled into a "nothing" model, in which no statistical information on any SNP could be reported. Given the current manner in which data protection is achieved and the existing protection technologies on the market, this is a logical situation. However, as recent research suggests, there is room to create a *gray* solution that resides within this policy space through the use of risk analysis strategies. Consider, as we mentioned above, if an adversary has access to summary information about a single SNP, then the likelihood the adversary can map an identified DNA sequence to the affected, nonaffected, or none of the above classes is significantly hampered. If provided with summary information about two SNPs, the probability that the adversary could link the identified record to one of the classes would be greater, but still extremely small. As we increase the number of SNPs that an investigator is permitted to have access to, the probability of linkage will increase. If data managers could determine the level of risk they are willing to tolerate, then they could disseminate information on a subset of SNPs consistent with their level of risk tolerance. This is precisely the basis for a formal and provable data protection strategy in accordance with the statistical data protection standard mentioned in the previous section.

RECOMMENDATIONS AND FUTURE DIRECTIONS

The above sections provided a high-level analysis of the existing threats and potential opportunities for OTRIS. This section formalizes specific recommendations regarding technologies and policies to improve data privacy protections. There is no single solution that will address all privacy and identifiability issues, but a combination of technical, policy, and legal mechanisms will help ameliorate potential problems.

As biomedical data sharing increases and systems move toward open access, there are certain guidelines and recommendations we believe OTRIS should consider. The following recommendations are briefly summarized in **Table 4-2**.

1. **Publishing aggregate statistical information for known replicable features only when the risk of exploiting such features is sufficiently low.** Given current NIH policies, it is recommended that OTRIS not post pooled statistical information regarding static, replicable features that are easy to derive from biological information, such as genome-wide SNP scans, on publicly accessible web servers. Though the risk of an individual actually applying such information in a linkage attack is unknown, the posting of such information will be in direct contradiction

T A B L E   **4-2** | **A Summary of Technical and Policy Approaches for OTRIS Data Privacy Protection**

1. Publish **aggregate statistics** of biomedical data **only when there is low risk** of exploiting the data for linkage.
2. Assess the **replication reliability** of molecular data
3. Define **access policies** and assess credentials of users
4. Define **use agreements**
5. Solicit **informed consent** for future data use when appropriate
6. Formalize **liability** and **redress** procedures
7. Establish **auditing** practices
8. Use multiple **levels of data detail** and oversight when possible
9. Adopt technically **formal reidentification risk mitigation** approaches (e.g., k-anonymity)

of policies adopted by similar NIH repositories and recent statements of the NIH director.[2]

2. **Assess the replicability of molecular data types.** As noted earlier, functional genomics data may be the focus of a given database repository. It is anticipated that the reliability of data replication will be data-type specific and it is thus recommended that OTRIS management discuss this issue with the scientists submitting data. If data are unreliably replicable, then the risk of publishing such information is less of a concern and the OTRIS may justify less strict oversight to access the data. If, on the other hand, such data are reliably replicable, then data in the OTRIS could be subject to a pool attack. In this case, it is recommended that such data should not be shared publicly.

3. **Establish polices for assessing credentials of data users and committees to institute the policies.** It is recommended that formal data access policies be established and published on the appropriate OTRIS management's website or made available through the appropriate regulatory bodies. In association with a formalized policy, it is further recommended that OTRIS establish a data access committee that reviews applications for access to data. This committee may be designed in a similar manner to the dbGaP DAC, but should be tailored to the needs of the repository. Individuals that serve on this committee could be drawn, to the extent it is possible, from the following classes:

   A. Ethicists
   B. Lawyers/counselors
   C. Scientists that deposited data into the OTRIS
   D. Program Managers from funding agencies, including
      i. Scientific Research Officials
      ii. Science Policy Officials

   Additional groups that may be represented on such a committee could consist of

   A. Patients/Community Advocates for whom data in the OTRIS corresponds
   B. External advisors from related biomedical repositories (e.g., dbGaP) or projects (e.g., the GAIN network (36), the eMERGE consortium (37))

   If the resource determines that data should be made available to anyone with a legitimate request, the access committee's role may only need to define what such requests correspond to and perform expedited reviews of requests for data access.

4. **Define use agreements.** It is recommended that the OTRIS determine what is considered acceptable use with respect to accessed data. Such information should be codified and explicitly defined in a data use contract that is agreed upon by the data recipient. It is recommended that the OTRIS work with legal experts with experience in this area to establish appropriate terms.

5. **Informed consent should describe, to the extent possible, the risks of data aggregation and reuse.** Deidentification and controlled access are essential aspects of legal and ethical data reuse from existing research databases and electronic health records. At the same time, however, much information will come from prospective

---

[2]There are emerging algorithms, implemented in working software, that can help data managers determine which features can be disclosed while ensuring that the probability of classifying an individual is below a predefined threshold. Yet, until such approaches are tied to appropriate policy models, their implementation will be limited.

mechanistic and translational studies, including GWAS. In these cases, the informed consent process must disclose the potential data sharing mechanisms described in this chapter. It should be recognized that it may not be possible to describe all of the future users of a subject's deidentified data, and it may not be legally possible for subjects to consent to unspecified future uses (38). However, subjects should be entitled with the opportunity to authorize future uses of their data for particular types of studies and withhold permission for others (39). Documentation of such understanding by subjects when they enter into research studies will assist Institutional Review Boards and Ethics Committees to provide the necessary certification when data are shared according to NIH policies. Moreover, clear demonstration that subjects in genetic research know and understand the potential of reidentification may lessen the regulation imposed in response to various privacy-invading mechanisms, such as the aforementioned pool attack.

6. **Formalize liability requirements and procedures for redress.** Though data shared through the OTRIS may be deidentified, it may be potentially reidentifiable. As such, the resource needs to determine the extent to which it is willing to assume liability for misuse of data. For instance, if a data user actually performs reidentification of a record, and such a reidentification becomes known, there should be a standing policy for how best to address and/or reprimand the user. Responding to the situation may be handled by the OTRIS itself, the user's home institution (if one exists), the originating institution of the data, or by any combination of the parties. Regardless, policies and procedures need to be established and agreed upon by all parties involved. Again, the resource should work with appropriate legal specialists and stakeholders in this activity.

7. **Establish auditing practices.** Even if the OTRIS chooses to make data "public" (or "semipublic"), it should enable auditing capability. In doing so, the OTRIS should assign unique login and passwords for each data user and log their activities in immutable audit logs. The resource should also determine when and how to audit users of the OTRIS. In most cases, data users will not act maliciously, but they may violate terms of service or best practices of use without realizing it.

8. **Consider multiple levels of accessibility and oversight to access information.** It is recommended that the managers of the OTRIS determine what they consider to be acceptable levels of risk and realistic vulnerabilities to the data in the system (the examples of high- and low-risk identifiers discussed earlier can help guide this discussion). If possible, the OTRIS may wish to provide access to different levels of data detail. For instance, it could provide access to aggregate statistics at one level and detailed microdata at another. At all levels, the aforementioned access committee should be involved. Moreover, it should be noted that managing aggregate statistical features of biological or molecular data in the same manner as the actual microdata is an overprotective and potentially research-limiting step. For resources of lower risk (such as aggregates), the committee may choose to apply expedited reviews to ensure that the requests are in line with acceptable use policies, similar to those applied by Institutional Review Boards (IRBs). The goal is to minimize the amount of time that the committee needs to spend reviewing an individual's request to access data. In contrast, for access to more detailed information, the committee may use a more stringent review process and require additional restrictions on data access and transferability.

If aggregate statistics are to be made available, it should be recognized that there is no universal solution to mitigate identifiability. There is no definite set of data attributes that, if suppressed, will guarantee protection from the data being reidentified. Rather, it is recommended that risk estimates be performed to determine the level of risk involved with sharing the data (note—this risk is data and not attribute dependent), and these risks should be deemed acceptable to the data managers, whether it is the investigators sharing data to the OTRIS, the sponsoring agency's program managers, or OTRIS administrators.

9. **Adopt technical approaches to mitigate reidentification risk.** As mentioned earlier, different types of data lead to different linkage concerns. Some data can be linked to publicly available data—especially demographics. It should be recognized that even if data shared via a database resource adheres to HIPAA Safe Harbor levels of protection, there is no guarantee the data are impregnable to reidentification. Thus, if there is concern that someone would attempt to discredit the OTRIS by identifying a single record in the database, then managers should consider disclosing data according to a more formal data protection model. One manner by which the OTRIS can formally mitigate risk is to generalize and/or suppress data to ensure that each record corresponds to a certain number of people (i.e., a minimum bin size).

Technically, the resource may consider a formal protection model, such as k-anonymity (40). In this model, the data protector chooses a k that specifies the risk deemed to be acceptable; specifically, k corresponds to how many people data managers want each specific record to link to. The question remains, however, of what is the appropriate level of k to be chosen. For some guidance, the various statistical agencies have suggested that around five appears to be an acceptable solution. Whether this is directly applicable to life sciences data remains an open question. If deemed acceptable, this is a solution that can be tailored to any dataset in an OTRIS. In other words, k could be made dependent on the "sensitivity" of the data in question or the amount of harm that could be committed through the data.

The benefits of a privacy model, such as k-anonymity, are that it (i) appears to satisfy the HIPAA protection policy of the statistic or scientific standard and (ii) requires the data holder to cognitively be involved in the protection of data. The drawbacks are that (a) it is not clear how k-anonymization affects the utility of the data for translational hypothesis generation and data mining in particular and (b) it is not clear how k-anonymized data can be analyzed with typical statistical packages, let alone specialized software for complex data types. Nonetheless, many biomedical research studies are concerned with the discovery, or application, of common genetic and clinical variants, such that a formal data protection model may sufficiently preserve enough biomedical information for future investigators. Additional research is necessary to determine when this technical method of data protection is applicable.

The policy and technology recommendations outlined above can be combined for flexible control. The recommendations should be used as the OTRIS deems necessary. The main goal is to strike an appropriate balance, where the technical aspects of data protection are complemented with acceptable use and oversight policies. If data users are more trusted, then data may be disseminated in a more specific form with stringent use contracts and if users are deemed to be less trusted, then data may be disclosed in more aggregated form with weaker use contracts.

CONCLUSIONS

In conclusion, there is increasing awareness by all of the various stakeholders involved in human studies research—research sponsors, investigators and subject participants—that in order to maximize the return on the investment that all parties make in clinical research it is advantageous to make the results widely available to the research community. A variety of OTRIS resources have been established to facilitate the sharing and reuse of these valuable data. However, while the benefits of data sharing are recognized, the requirements for maintaining the autonomy, privacy, and confidentiality of the research participants must also be addressed. We have presented a series of recommendations regarding both technical and policy approaches designed to minimize the risk of participant reidentification from clinical research data. By adopting these recommendations, OTRIS can balance the benefits gained by data sharing while minimizing the risk to the research participants.

ACKNOWLEDGMENTS

The authors wish to thank Dr. Ellen Wright Clayton of Vanderbilt University, Jeff Wiser of Northrop Grumman, and the anonymous referees for helpful discussions and recommendations regarding the writing of this chapter. Supported by the following grants from the US National Institutes of Health: N01AI40076, R01LM009989, U01HG004603, UL1RR023468, and UL1RR024982.

REFERENCES

1. Kaiser J. Biobanks: population databases boom, from Iceland to the US. *Science.* 2002;298:1158–1161.
2. Kaye J, Heeney C, Hawkins N, et al. Data sharing and genomics—reshaping scientific practices. *Nat Rev Genet.* 2009;10:331–335.
3. Piwowar H, Becich M, Bilofsky H, et al. Towards a data sharing culture: recommendations for leadership from academic health centers. *PLoS Med.* 2008;5:e183.
4. Karp D, Carlin S, Cook-Deegan R, et al. Ethical and practical issues associated with aggregating databases. *PLoS Med.* 2008;5:e190.
5. McGuire A, Caulfield T, Cho M. Research ethics and the challenge of whole-genome sequencing. *Nat Rev Genet.* 2008;9(2):152–156.
6. Malin B. An evaluation of the current state of genomic data privacy protection technology and a roadmap for the future. *J Am Med Inform Assoc.* 2005;12:28–34.
7. Homer N, Szelinger S, Redman M, et al. Resolving individuals contributing trace amounts of DNA to highly complex mixtures using high-density SNP genotyping microarrays. *PLoS Genet.* 2008;4:e1000167.
8. Sankararaman S, Obozinksi G, Jordan M, et al. Genomic privacy and limits of individual detection in a pool. *Nat Genet.* 2009;41:965–967.
9. Mailman M, Feolo M, Jin Y, et al. The NCBI database of genotypes and phenotypes. *Nat Genet.* 2007;39:1181–1186.
10. Zerhouni E, Nabel E. Protecting aggregate genomic data. *Science.* 2008;322:44.

11. National Institutes of Health. Final NIH statement on sharing research data. NOT-OD-03-032. February 26, 2003.

12. National Institutes of Health. Policy for sharing of data obtained in NIH supported or conducted genome-wide association studies (GWAS). Notice NOT-OD-07-088. August 28, 2007.

13. U.S. Department of Health and Human Services. Standards for privacy of individually identifiable health information, Final Rule. 45 CFR, Parts 160–164. *Fed. Regist.* 2002;67(157):53182–53273.

14. Gostin L, Nass S. Reforming the HIPAA privacy rule: safeguarding privacy and promoting research. *JAMA.* 2009;301:1373–1375.

15. National Association of Health Data Organizations. NAHDO Inventory of State-wide Hospital Discharge Data Activities. Falls Church, VA: National Association of Health Data Organizations; 2008.

16. Schoenman J, Sutton J, Kintala S, et al. The value of hospital discharge databases: final report to the Agency for Healthcare Research and Quality under contract number 282-98-0024 (task order number 5). *White paper, NORC at the University of Chicago, in cooperation with the National Association of Health data Organizations.* 2005. Available at http://www.hcup-us.ahrq.gov/reports/final_report.pdf. Accessed August 8, 2009.

17. Brawley S. Submission and retrieval of an aligned set of nucleic acid sequences. *J Phycol.* 1999;35:433–437.

18. Lin Z, Hewett M, Altman R. Using binning to maintain confidentiality of medical data. *Proc AMIA Symp.* 2002;454–458.

19. Lin Z, Owen A, Altman R. Genetics: genomic research and human subject privacy. *Science.* 2004;305:183.

20. Kargupta H, Datta S, Wang Q, et al. Random-data perturbation techniques and privacy-preserving data mining. *Knowl Inf Syst.* 2005;7:387–414.

21. Sweeney L. Weaving technology and policy together to maintain confidentiality. *J Law Med Ethics.* 1997;25:98–110.

22. Golle P. Revisiting the uniqueness of simple demographics in the U.S. population. In *Proceedings of the 2006 ACM Workshop on Privacy in the Electronic Society,* 2006:77–80.

23. Sweeney L. Uniqueness of simple demographics in the US population. *White Paper LIDAP-WP4,* Laboratory for International Data Privacy, Carnegie Mellon University. 2000.

24. Loukides G, Denny J, Malin B. Do clinical profiles constitute privacy risks? *Proc AMIA Symp.* 2009: to appear.

25. Malin B. Re-identification of familial database records. *Proc AMIA Symp.* 2006:524–528.

26. Malin B, Sweeney L. How (not) to protect genomic data privacy in a distributed network: using trail re-identification to evaluate and design anonymity protection systems. *J Biomed Inform.* 2004;37:179–192.

27. Altman R, Klein T. Challenges for biomedical informatics and pharmacogenomics. *Annu Rev Pharmacol Toxicol.* 2002;42:113–133.

28. De Moor G, Claerhout B, De Meyer F. Privacy enhancing techniques: the key to secure communication and management of clinical and genomic data. *Methods Inf Med.* 2003;42:148–153.

29. Dugas M, Schoch C, Schnittger S, et al. Impact of integrating clinical and genetic information. *In Silico Biol.* 2002;2:383–391.

30. Sweeney L. Guaranteeing anonymity when sharing medical data, the Datafly system. *Proc AMIA Symp.* 1997:51–55.

31. Malin B. Betrayed by my shadow: learning data identity via trail matching. *J Privacy Technol.* 2005;2005:0609001.

32. Aldhous P. Genetic data withdrawn amid privacy concerns. *New Scientist.* September 1, 2008.

33. Clabby C. DNA research commons scaled back. *Am Sci.* 2009;97(2):113.

34. Ferris N. The search for John Doe. *Government Health IT Magazine.* January 26, 2009.

35. Patoine B. Nervecenter: speed bump for open access to genomic data. *Ann Neurol.* 2008;64:A16–A17.

36. Manolio T, Rodriguez LL, Brooks L, et al. New models of collaboration in genome-wide association studies: the Genetic Association Information Network. GAIN Collaborative Research Group. *Nat Genet.* 2007;39:1045–1051.

37. Manolio T. Collaborative genome-wide association studies of diverse diseases: programs of the NHGRI's office of population genomics. *Pharmacogenomics.* 2009;10:235–241.

38. Greely H. The uneasy ethical and legal underpinnings of large-scale genomic biobioanks. *Annu Rev Genomics Hum Genet.* 2007;8:343–364.

39. Caulfield T, Upshur, R, Daar A. DNA databanks and consent: a suggested policy option involving an authorization model. *BMC Med Ethics.* 2003;4:1.

40. Sweeney L. K-anonymity: a model for protecting privacy. *Int J Uncertain Fuzz.* 2002;10:557–570.

CHAPTER 5

Writing a Statistical Analysis Plan

Beverley Adams-Huet, MS and Chul Ahn, PhD

INTRODUCTION

Clinical research is judged to be valid not by the results but how it is designed and conducted. The cliché of "do it right or do it over" is particularly apt in clinical research.

One of the questions a clinical investigator frequently asks in planning clinical research is "Do I need a statistician as part of my clinical research team?" The answer is "Yes!" since a statistician can help to optimize design, analysis and interpretation of results, and drawing conclusions. When developing a clinical research proposal, how early in the process should the clinical investigator contact the statistician? Answer—it is never too early. Statistics cannot rescue a poorly designed protocol after the study has begun. A statistician can be a valuable member of a clinical research team and often serves as a coinvestigator. Large multicenter projects, such as Phase III randomized clinical trials for drug approval by a regulatory agency, nearly always have a statistician (or several) on their team. However, smaller, typically single-center studies may also require rigorous statistical methodology in design and analysis. These studies are often devised by young clinical investigators launching their clinical research career who may have not collaborated with a statistician. Many clinical investigators are familiar with the statistical role in the analysis of research data (1), but researchers may not be aware of the role of a statistician in designing clinical research and developing the study protocol. In this chapter, we discuss topics and situations that clinical investigators and statisticians commonly encounter while planning a research study and writing the statistical methods section. We stress the importance of having the statistical methodology planned well in advance of conducting the clinical research study. Working in conjunction with a statistician can also be a key training opportunity for the clinical investigator beginning a clinical research career.

GETTING STARTED ON THE STATISTICAL ANALYSIS PLAN

Why work with a statistician? The study design, sample size, and statistical analysis must be able to properly evaluate the research hypothesis set forth by the clinical investigator. Otherwise, the consequences of a poorly developed statistical approach may result in a failure to obtain extramural funding and result in a flawed clinical study that cannot adequately test the desired hypotheses. Statisticians provide design advice and develop the statistical methods that best correspond to the research hypothesis. For the planning of a clinical study, a statistician can provide valuable information on key design points as summarized in **Table 5-1**. The statistician can discuss with the clinical investigators questions such as: Is the design valid? Overly ambitious? Will the data be analyzable?

Very early in the planning stages, it is important to send the statistician a draft of the proposal. Any protocol changes may affect the required sample size and analysis plans, and so it is important to meet with the statistician throughout the planning stages and later if modifications have been made to the study design. Before the statistical section can be

TABLE **5-1** | The Role of the Statistician in Developing the Statistical Plan

- Clarify the research questions or hypothesis. Are the primary hypotheses clearly stated, adequate, and realistic?
- Identify the outcome variables related to the research questions. Are the primary or secondary endpoints clearly defined?
- Does the study design appropriately and adequately address the proposed hypothesis?
- Are the issues of the bias, blinding, or stratification properly handled in the study?
- Are the assumptions used for sample size estimation clearly elaborated and supported by proper preliminary data and/or references?
- Is there a clearly specified, appropriate data analysis plan?
- Is there an appropriate data and safety monitoring plan, interim analysis plan, or preestablished early stopping rule?

RESEARCH ETHICS: PITFALLS & PRESCRIPTIONS

From an IRB and research ethics perspective, good research design and statistical power define the scientific benefits that justify the risks to research participants. If your design is seriously flawed or your data analysis is invalid, then your study cannot be ethically justified nor approved by an IRB.

Wendler D, Miller FG. Risk-benefit analysis and the net risks test. In: Emanuel EJ, Grady C, Crouch RA, et al., eds. *The Oxford Textbook of Clinical Research Ethics.* New York: Oxford University Press; 2008:503–513.

developed, what information does the statistician need? Questions from a statistician concerning design, power and sample size, and analysis may include:

- What is the research hypothesis?
- What is the type of study design?
- What is the most important measurement (primary outcome variable)?
- What is the type of variable and unit of measurement?
- What is a clinically meaningful difference for the primary outcome?
- How many subjects can be recruited or observed within a study period? How many groups or treatment arms are to be included in your design?
- Will there be an equal number of participants or observations in each group? That is, what is the allocation ratio?
- How many total evaluations and measurements?
- For repeated measurements, what is the measurement interval?

You are not expected to have all the answers at your first meeting, and ongoing conversations with the statistician can serve to develop these ideas. Eventually, the answers to these questions comprise the justification for the design selected, provide the basis for the sample size estimate, and drive the choice of statistical analysis. A brief consultation with a statistician will not be adequate to address these issues. The interaction with a statistician to construct the statistical section is not usually one meeting, email, or phone call. It is a process that will help you think through the design of your study. This is also an excellent opportunity to ask questions and enhance your statistical education. Additionally, the exchange of ideas is beneficial to the statistician who will better appreciate the clinical research question. The discussions with a statistician could lead to changes in study design, such as proposing a smaller, more focused study design to collect preliminary data.

A general outline of the statistical methods section is shown in **Table 5-2**. There may be deviations from this format depending on the particular study design. The statistical write-up is rarely less than one page and may total several pages. Although some clinical investigators trained in statistics do prepare this section, more commonly the statistician constructs and writes up the statistical methods section for grants and protocols in close collaboration with the investigators. However, it is important that clinical investigators develop a conceptual understanding of the proposed statistical methodology. Take advantage of any study design and biostatistics classes offered at your institutions to make statistical collaborations more fruitful.

T A B L E **5-2** | Outline of the Statistical Methods Section

I. Study design
  • Type of design
  • Sampling
  • Power and sample size
  • Randomization and blinding
II. Statistical analysis methodology
  • Define data analysis set
  • Statistical analysis
    i. Primary analysis
    ii. Secondary analysis
    iii. Exploratory
  • Missing data
  • Multiplicity of testing
  • Subgroup analyses, covariates
  • Interim analysis

STUDY DESIGN

Type of Design

Before the statistical section can progress, the study design must be known. Study designs that are commonly used in clinical research include case–control, cohort, randomized controlled design, crossover, and factorial designs. A randomized controlled trial has many features but most commonly incorporates what is called a parallel group design where individuals are randomly assigned to a particular treatment or intervention group. In a crossover study, the subject participates in more than one study intervention phase, ideally studied in a random sequence, such as comparing triglyceride responses within the same individual on a low-fat versus a high-fat diet.

Sampling

How do we select participants for the study? There are many types of sampling procedures, the basis of which is to avoid or reduce bias. Bias can be defined as "a systematic tendency to produce an outcome that differs from the underlying truth" (2). Although true randomness is the goal of a sampling, it is generally not achievable. The study subjects are not usually selected at random to participate in clinical research. Instead, in most clinical trials, the "random" element in randomization is that the consented subjects are assigned by chance to a particular treatment or intervention. The clinical inclusion and exclusion criteria coupled with informed consent will determine who will be the study participants and, ultimately, to what population the study results will be generalizable.

T A B L E **5-3** | Definitions for Statistical Hypothesis Testing

* A Type I error (α) is the risk of inferring a difference between study groups when there is no such difference.
* A Type II error (β) is the risk of inferring no difference between study groups when there is such a difference.
* Power is the statistical test's ability to detect a true difference. Power = 1-Type II error.

Sample Size

With the study design and the makeup of the study sample determined, the sample size estimates can be obtained. Fundamental to estimating sample size are the concepts of statistical hypothesis testing, Types I and II errors, and power **(Table 5-3)**. In planning clinical research, it is necessary to determine the number of subjects required so that the study achieves sufficient statistical power to detect the hypothesized effect. If the reader is not familiar with the concept of statistical hypothesis testing, introductory biostatistics texts, and many websites cover this topic (15). Briefly, in trials to demonstrate improved efficacy of a new treatment over placebo/standard treatments, the null hypothesis is that there is no difference between treatments and the alternative hypothesis is that there is a treatment difference. The research hypothesis usually corresponds to the alternative hypothesis, which represents a minimal meaningful difference in clinical outcomes. Statistically, we either reject the null hypothesis in favor of the alternative hypothesis or fail to reject the null hypothesis.

Typically, the sample size is computed to provide a fixed level of power under a specified alternative hypothesis. Power is an important consideration for several reasons. Low power can cause a true difference in clinical outcomes between study groups to go undetected. However, too much power may yield statistically significant results that are not meaningfully different to clinicians. The probability of Type I error (α) of 0.05 (two sided) and power of 0.80 and 0.90 have been widely used for the sample size estimation in clinical trials. The sample size estimate will also allow the estimation of the total cost of the proposed study.

A clinical trial that is conducted without attention to sample size or power information takes the risks of either failing to detect clinically meaningful differences (Type II error) due to not enough subjects or taking an unnecessarily excessive number of samples for a study. Both cases fail to adhere to the Ethical Guidelines of the American Statistical Association, which says "Avoid the use of excessive or inadequate number of research subjects by making informed recommendations for study size" (3).

What Information is Needed to Calculate Power and Sample Size?

The components that most sample size programs require for input include:

* Choose Type I error (α)
* Choose power
* Choose clinical outcome variable and effect size (difference between means, proportions, survival times, and regression parameters)

- Variation estimate
- Allocation ratio

Clinical Outcome Measures

Clearly describe the clinical outcomes that will be analyzed to the statistician. The variable type **(Table 5-4)** and distribution of the primary outcome measurement must be defined before sample size and power calculations can proceed. The sample size estimates are mainly needed for the primary outcome. However, providing power estimates for secondary outcomes is often helpful to reviewers.

Effect Size

As an example, suppose a parallel group study is being designed to compare systolic blood pressure between two treatments and the investigators want to be able to detect a mean 10 mm Hg difference between groups. This 10 mm Hg difference is referred to as the effect size, detectable difference, or minimal expected difference.

T A B L E   **5-4** | **Variable Types and Derivations to be Described in the Statistical Analysis Plan**

Describe each variable and type to be collected
- Categorical
  - Two categories (binary or dichotomous)
    - Sex (male, female), diabetes (Types I and II)
  - More than two categories
    - Blood type (O, A, B, and AB)
- Ordinal
  - Attitudes (strongly disagree, disagree, neutral, agree, and strongly agree)
  - Cancer stage (I, II, III, and IV)
- Survival (time to event)
  - Transplant free survival time
  - Time free from infection
- Numerical
  - Discrete
    - Number of abnormal cells
  - Continuous
    - Age
    - Serum creatinine
    - Log_e triglycerides (nonnormally distributed, log transformed due to skewness)
- Derived variables
  - Absolute and percent change
  - Area under the curve (AUC)
    - Insulin AUC from an oral glucose tolerance test
    - Receiver operating characteristic curve (ROC)
  - Pharmacokinetic parameters

How is the Effect Size Determined?

Choose an effect size that is based on clinical knowledge of the primary endpoint. A sample size that "worked" in a published paper is no guarantee of success in a different setting. The selected effect size is unique to your study intervention, the specific type of participants in your study sample, and perhaps an aspect of the outcome measurement that is unique to your clinic or laboratory (4).

The investigator and statistician examine the literature, the investigator's own past research, or a combination of the above to determine a study effect size. To investigate the difference in mean blood pressure between two treatments, the effect size options might be 2, 6, 10, or 20 mm Hg. Which of these differences do you need to have the ability to detect? **This is a clinical question, not a statistical question.** Effect size is a measure of the magnitude of the treatment effect and represents a clinically or biologically important difference. Choosing a 20-mm Hg effect size yields a smaller sample size than a 10-mm Hg effect size since it is easier to statistically detect the larger difference. However, an effect size of 10 mm Hg or smaller magnitude may be more a realistic treatment effect and less likely to result in a flawed or wasted study.

Variation Estimates for Sample Size Calculations

In addition to effect size, we may need to estimate how much the outcome varies from person to person. For continuous variables, the variation estimate is often in the form of a standard deviation. If the hypothesized difference in systolic blood pressure is an effect size of 10 mm Hg, a study with a blood pressure standard deviation of 22 mm Hg will have lower power than a study where the standard deviation is 14 mm Hg. For a continuous outcome such as blood pressure, a measure of the variation is another part of the formula needed to compute the sample size. An estimate of variation can be derived from a literature search or from the investigator's preliminary data. Obtaining this information can be a challenge for both the clinical investigator and statistician.

Table 5-5 shows sample sizes scenarios for detecting differences in blood pressure when comparing two treatment means based on a *t*-test. A standard deviation of 14 mm Hg is chosen

T A B L E **5-5** | Scenarios for Choosing Sample Size

Primary outcome variable	Effect size, mean detectable difference between groups	Estimated standard deviation[a]	Sample size per group[b], $\alpha = 0.05$	
			Power = 0.80	Power = 0.90
Blood pressure				
Systolic blood	6	14	86	115
pressure, mm Hg	8	14	49	65
	10	14	32	42
	20	14	9	11

[a]Estimates are derived from Ref. 5.
[b]The software used for the computations is the PS program developed by Dupont and Plummer (6).

to estimate the variation. Sample sizes are calculated for power of 0.80 and 0.90 at the two-sided 0.05-significance level. Notice that the smaller effect sizes require a larger sample size and that the sample size increases as the power increases from 0.80 to 0.90.

Determining a reasonable and affordable sample size estimate is a team effort. There are practical issues such as budgets or recruitment limitations that may come into play. A too large sample size could preclude the ability to conduct the research. The research team will assess scenarios with varying detectable differences and power as seen in **Table 5-5** (calculations performed using PS power (6) available at the website http://biostat.mc. vanderbilt.edu/twiki/bin/view/Main/PowerSampleSize). Typically, a scenario can be worked out that is both clinically and statistically viable.

The elements of sample size calculations presented here pertain to relatively simple designs. Cluster samples or family data need special statistical adjustments. For a longitudinal or repeated measures design, the correlation between the repeated measurements is incorporated into the sample size calculations (7,8).

Do All Studies Need Sample Size and Power Estimates?

Pilot Studies

Pilot studies may not need a power analysis since they are more about testing the protocol than testing a hypothesis (9). Sometimes there are no preliminary data, and thus pilot data must be obtained to provide estimates for designing for a more definitive study. However, calling a study a pilot study to avoid power analyses and to keep the sample small is misrepresentation (9).

Precision

Sample size calculations are necessary when the study goal is precision instead of power. The goal may be to describe the precision of a proportion or mean or other statistic that is to be estimated from our sample. Precision in this context is based on finding a suitably narrow confidence interval for the statistic of interest, such that the lower and upper limits of the confidence interval include a *clinically* meaningful range of values. We may want to know how many subjects are required to be 95% confident that an interval contains the true, but unknown, value. For example, how many subjects are needed for 10% precision if we expect a 30% allele prevalence in a genetic study? Instead of power, we estimate the sample size for the desired precision based on a single proportion of 0.30 and summarize by stating "With 80 subjects, the precision for a 30% allele prevalence rate is approximately 10% (95% confidence interval: 21% to 40%)." If greater precision is desirable then the sample size is increased accordingly.

Accounting for Attrition

Withdrawal and dropout are unwelcome realities of clinical research. Missing data in clinical trials or repeated measurement studies are inevitable. Consider missing data issues when designing, planning, and conducting studies to minimize missing data impact. Sample size estimates are finalized by adjusting for attrition based on the anticipated number of dropouts.

Randomization Plan

Random allocation of subjects to study groups is fundamental to the clinical trial design. Randomization, which is a way to reduce bias, involves random allocation of the participants to the treatment groups. If investigators compare a new treatment against a standard treatment, the study subjects are allocated to one of these treatments by a random process. A general description of the randomization approach may be introduced in the clinical methods section of the proposal, for example, "Treatment assignment will be determined using stratified, blocked randomization." Specific randomization details will need to be elaborated on in the statistical methods section, including how the allocation procedure will be implemented, for example, via computer programs, website, lists, or sealed envelopes. If stratification is deemed necessary, include in the proposal a description of each stratification variable and the number of levels for each stratum, for instance, gender (male, female), diabetes (type I, type II), etc. However, keep the number of strata and stratum levels minimal (10). Discuss the advantages and disadvantages of the various allocation approaches with the study statistician.

Blinding

Knowledge of the treatment assignment might influence how much of a dosage change is made to a study treatment or how an adverse event is assessed. Blinding or masking is another component of study design used to try to eliminate such bias (11). In a double-blind randomized trial, neither the study subjects nor the clinical investigators know the treatment assignment.

Describe the planned blinding scheme. For example, "This is a double-blind randomized study to investigate the effect of propranolol versus no propranolol on the incidences of total mortality and of total mortality plus nonfatal myocardial infarction in 158 older patients with CHF and prior myocardial infarction." Specify who is to be blinded and the steps that will be taken to maintain the blind. It is important that evaluators such as a radiologists, pathologists, or lab personnel who have no direct contact with the study subjects remain blinded to treatment assignments.

It may be impossible or difficult to use the double-blind procedures in some clinical trials. For example, it is not feasible to design a double-blind clinical trial for the comparison of surgical and nonsurgical interventions. Or, blinding might not be completely successful; study personnel may be inadvertently alerted as to the probable treatment assignment due to the occurrence of a specific adverse event. If blinding is not feasible, offer an explanation for lack of blinding procedures in the research proposal.

STATISTICAL ANALYSIS METHODOLOGY

The statistical analysis methods for analyzing the study outcomes are to be carefully detailed. Specifying these methods in advance is another way to minimize bias and maintain the integrity of the analysis. Any changes to the statistical methods must be justified and decided on before the blind is broken (12). In the statistical analysis plan not only must the statistical hypotheses to be tested be described and justified but also detail which subjects and observations will be included or excluded in each analysis.

TABLE **5-6** | Analysis Data Sets

Intention-to-treat principle—the principle that asserts that the effect of a treatment policy can be best assessed by evaluating on the basis of the intention to treat a subject (i.e., the planned treatment regimen) rather than the actual treatment given. It has the consequence that subjects allocated to a treatment group should be followed up, assessed, and analyzed as members of that group irrespective of their compliance with the planned course of treatment.

Full analysis data set—the set of subjects that is as close as possible to the ideal implied by the intention-to-treat principle. It is derived from the set of all randomized subjects by minimal and justified elimination of subjects.

Per protocol data set (valid cases, efficacy sample, and evaluable subject's sample)— the set of data generated by the subset of subjects who complied with the protocol sufficiently to ensure that these data would be likely to exhibit the effects of treatment according to the underlying scientific model. Compliance covers such considerations as exposure to treatment, availability of measurements, and absence of major protocol violations.

From ICH E9: Guidance for Industry—E9 Statistical Principles for Clinical Trials, U.S. Department of Health and Human Services, Food and Drug Administration, September 1998 (12). Available at: http://www.fda.gov/downloads/RegulatoryInformation/Guidances/UCM129505.pdf.

Analysis Data Sets

Intention-to-Treat Analysis

It is crucial to define the primary sample of subjects analyzed in the reporting of clinical trial results. Defined in **Table 5-6**, intention-to-treat (ITT) and per protocol analyses are commonly reported in medical literature result sections. For a randomized study, ITT analysis is the gold standard for the primary analysis and the ITT principle is regarded as the most appropriate criteria for the assessment of a new therapy by the Food and Drug Administration and the National Institute of Health (13). An ITT data set includes all randomized subjects, whether or not they were compliant or completed the study. Adhering to the ITT principle mirrors what occurs in clinical practice where a patient may discontinue a medication or miss a clinic appointment. This avoids biases that can result from dropouts and missing data. However, the missing data must not bias the treatment comparisons (14), otherwise the statistics may not be valid. This type of bias could occur if the dropouts or missed study visits are related to a particular treatment group and are not observed equally across all of the treatments.

A true ITT data set may not be attainable in all clinical trials. There might be no postrandomization or posttreatment data for a study subject who withdraws from the study at the initial study visit. Then the primary analysis might consist of all subjects who took at least one treatment dose or had at least one follow-up visit (12). Anticipate these possibilities as the study is designed and specify in the statistical analysis plan that subjects and observations will comprise the "full analysis set." Prespecification of these data sets prior to statistical analysis is imperative.

Per protocol Analysis

It may be of clinical interest to plan an analysis set that consists of only "completers" or "compliers." A per protocol analysis, defined in **Table 5-6**, is more likely to be planned as secondary analyses. If the per protocol analysis results are not consistent with the ITT analysis results, then closely examine the reasons behind any discrepancy.

Statistical Analysis

The statistical analysis plan is driven by the research questions, the study design, and the type of the outcome measurements. The analysis plan includes a detailed description of statistical testing for each of the variables in the Specific Aim(s). If several Specific Aims are proposed, we write an analysis plan for each Specific Aim. Plan descriptive analyses for each group or planned subgroup. If subjects were randomly assigned to groups, it is expected that there will be a description of subject characteristics that include demographic information as well as baseline measurements or comorbid conditions. Specify anticipated data transformations that may be needed to meet analysis assumptions and describe derived variables to be created such as area under the curve. Incorporate confidence intervals in the analysis plan for reporting treatment effects. Confidence limits are much more informative to the reader than are p-values alone (15).

Statistical details and terminology are not intended to be an obstacle for a young investigator. Instead this is where the statistical expert can be a valuable resource to help the investigators use the appropriate statistical methods and language that address the research hypotheses. Brief statistical analysis descriptions are shown in **Table 5-7** for a randomized study and a longitudinal cohort study. In addition to the general methodology of **Table 5-7**, we explain in the statistical methods section how statistical assumptions or model diagnostics will be evaluated. Describe the hypotheses to be tested with the corresponding statistical tests for the primary, secondary, and exploratory analyses. In the medical literature, statistical analyses such as chi-square and t-tests, analysis of variance, regression modeling, and various nonparametric tests are common. However, the statistician is happy to advise whether these traditional methods are appropriate for the research question at hand or if other approaches would be more suitable.

Statistics, like medicine, is a large and diverse field; hence statisticians have specific areas of expertise. Some proposals may require one statistician for the design and analysis of medical imaging studies and another statistician for design and analysis of a microarray study. Often a proposal specifies one statistician as the study statistician and another statistician to serve on a Data and Safety Monitoring Board.

Interim Analysis

Conducting a planned interim analysis in an ongoing clinical trial can be beneficial for scientific, economic, and ethical reasons (16). Formal interim analyses include stopping rules for terminating the study early if a treatment shows futility or clear benefit or harm. The termination of the estrogen plus progestin treatment arm of the Women's Health Initiative clinical trial in 2002 (17) when the treatment risks exceeded benefits demonstrates the strong clinical impact of interim analyses. However, interim analyses are not to be undertaken lightly. Taking unplanned repeated looks at accumulating data is problematic. First, it raises the multiple testing issue so that adjustments to control the overall Type I error rate are necessary. Second, the results can interfere with the conduct of the remainder of the study, creating bias. Pocock (18) and O'Brien and Fleming (19) authored the

TABLE **5-7** | Statistical Analysis Plans

A. Statistical analysis example for a randomized study
Statistical analysis: The full analysis set will include patients who have received at least one dose of medication or had one or more postrandomization, follow-up evaluation. Descriptive statistics will be computed for each treatment group, Medians and percentiles will be reported for skewed continuous variables. For primary and secondary outcomes, descriptive statistics and 95% confidence intervals will used to summarize the differences between groups. The primary outcome of systolic blood pressure and other continuous variables will be assessed with a repeated measures analysis using a mixed linear model approach. Since many of the inflammatory markers are positively skewed, interleukin-6 and c-reactive protein will be log transformed prior to analysis. The Wilcoxon Rank Sum test will be used to compare pill counts between groups. Hypothesis tests will be two sided using the 0.05-significance level. Bonferroni type adjustments for multiple testing will be implemented to control Type I errors. Statistical analysis will be performed with SAS software (SAS Institute, Cary, NC, USA).

B. Statistical analysis example for a longitudinal cohort study
Descriptive/comparative statistics defining the biomarker levels in the different disease activity classes. We will compute and compare the mean/median, and interquartile range of urine biomarker levels in different disease activity groups, after partitioning patients in various ways: patients who attain any of the primary disease outcomes, that is, WHO Class IIII or IV glomerulonephritis, patients with nephritic or nephrotic flares, or end-stage renal disease. Additionally, we will define the biomarker levels in patients with the following disease features: anemia, leucopenia, or thrombocytopenia. For comparing multiple patient groups, analysis of variance (ANOVA) or the Kruskal–Wallis test will be used, depending on whether the biomarker values are normally distributed. Data transformations will be performed if necessary. If the omnibus ANOVA or Kruskal–Wallis test yields $p < 0.05$, we will conduct pairwise group comparisons using either t-tests or Wilcoxon Rank Sum tests with Bonferroni corrections. The generalized estimating equations (GEE) approach will be used to evaluate if urinary biomarkers vary significantly over time among different disease activity classes.

classic approaches for defining statistical stopping rules. The alpha spending function described by DeMets and Lan (20) provides some flexibility for the timing of interim analyses as well as controlling the Type I error rate. Clinical investigators must seriously consider what decisions might have to be made based on interim analysis results and how this will affect an ongoing study.

OVERLOOKED AREAS

Matching in Case–Control Studies

A weakness that often surfaces in sessions reviewing research proposals is an inadequate description of matching. Matching is commonly used in case–control studies by selecting for each case a control with the same value of the confounding variable. However, in our experience, the term "matching" is used too loosely. To a reviewer matching implies the recruitment of matched pairs. This may not be the intention of the investigators or the planned statistical analysis approach. A proposal that states that the participants will be matched according to the gender, race/ethnicity, age, and body mass index would raise quite a few questions because "matching" on all these variables would be quite difficult to achieve in practice. Often what the investigator really would like to insure is that the study groups will be balanced with respect to these characteristics. This is described as "frequency matching." For continuous variables, such as age, the range that is considered a "match" needs to be specified. Indicate the target age range that is clinically comparable for your study, for example, within 2 or 5 years. Avoid matching on variables that are not known confounders as this may lead to loss of power (21).

Missing Data Prevention

It is well known that dropouts and certain missing data patterns can impact a study's validity. Since statistical analyses cannot cure all problems associated with missing data, prevention is the best policy. To minimize dropouts and missed study visits, verify that the proposal has included a retention plan. Incorporate study procedures that may help to reduce the amount of missing data, such as making regular calls to participants to better maintain contact as the study is underway (see Chapter 8 for detailed approaches to study subject retention). Every member of the research team must appreciate the need to reschedule or repeat key study visits or labs to the extent possible if the primary outcome measurement was not obtained. In order to obtain an analysis set that is consistent with the ITT principle, continue to schedule follow-up visits and collect primary outcome measurements for subjects who have discontinued their assigned treatment.

Database

The integrity of the statistical analysis depends on the quality of the data. Obviously a study must contain high-quality data (garbage in, garbage out), but steps to ensure this are frequently overlooked. Describe in the research proposal how data will be collected, deidentified, stored, and protected. It is vital that the clinical research team becomes skilled at data management. Meet with a database expert early to discuss the design of a database and related forms and involve the statistician in the review of the forms. Development of the proper data forms and database prior to study activation is essential.

DISCUSSION

We have presented guidance to be considered when developing the statistical plan in proposals for clinical and translational research. All these approaches have the common theme of eliminating or reducing bias and improving study quality. Planning the statistical methodology in advance is crucial for maintaining the integrity of clinical research. We hope we have conveyed that developing the statistical methods for a research proposal is a collaborative effort between statistical and clinical research professionals.

Writing the statistical plan is a multidisciplinary effort. Both the clinical investigator and statistician on the research team need to carefully review the final product and ensure that the science and statistics correspond correctly. Just as a statistician who can understand the clinical aspect of the research is particularly advantageous, endeavor to learn all you can from the statistical expert. Ask the statistician to explain the rationale of the statistical methodology so you can defend the statistical plans without the statistician at your side. The clinical investigator may not have to know how to perform complex analyses but does need to understand the general statistical reasoning behind the proposed statistical design and analysis. When clinical investigators have a basic proficiency in statistical methodology, not only are collaborations with statisticians more dynamic and fruitful but also the potential to develop into a strong, independent clinical investigator and mentor increases. This leads to the design and execution of more efficient and advanced research, increasing the productivity of the entire research team.

Statistical Resources and Education

What if the researcher does not have funding to support a biostatistician? One option is to include a biostatistician as a coinvestigator in your grant proposal to cover salary and supplies needed to implement the statistical methods described in the grant. Hopefully there is a department or division of Biostatistics or related field at your or a nearby institution. If not, long-distance collaborations can succeed via conference calls and email. The American Statistical Association (ASA) has an ASA consulting section (http://www.amstat.org/sections/cnsl/) where a clinical investigator can get assistance in finding a statistical consultant.

Some useful statistical websites for general statistical information and definitions include "The Little Handbook of Statistical Practice" (http://www.tufts.edu/~gdallal/LHSP.HTM); "HyperStat Online Statistics Textbook" (http://davidmlane.com/hyperstat/index.html); and WISE Web Interface for Statistical Education (http://wise.cgu.edu/index.html). Clinical trial statistical guidelines are documented in the International Conference on Harmonisation (ICH) Guidance for industry: E9 Statistical principles for clinical trials (http://www.fda.gov/) (12).

As of September 2009, 46 medical research institutions in the United States have been granted a Clinical and Translational Science Award (CTSA, http://www.ncrr.nih.gov/crctsa). When the CTSA program is fully implemented, it will support approximately 60 centers across the nation. Some CTSA awardees offer biostatistical collaboration or institutional pilot grants for early career clinical investigators in need of statistical expertise. Many of these research centers offer Biostatistics courses or seminar series that are specifically designed for clinical researchers. This chapter evolves from a CTSA course, "Clinical Research from Proposal to Implementation," taught at the University of Texas Southwestern at Dallas. Take advantage of any such course offerings and resources.

CONCLUSION

A successful research proposal requires solid statistical methodology. The written statistical methods section is the result of teamwork between the clinical investigators and statisticians. Collaborating with a statistician early and often will help the study proposal evolve into a strong application that increases opportunities for scientific acceptance and funding for conducting important clinical research studies.

REFERENCES

1. Altman DG, Goodman SN, Schroter S. How statistical expertise is used in medical research. *JAMA*. 2002;287:2817–2820.
2. Guyatt GH, Sackett DL, Cook DJ. Users' guides to the medical literature. II. How to use an article about therapy or prevention. A. Are the results of the study valid? Evidence-Based Medicine Working Group. *JAMA*. 1993;270:2598–2601.
3. American Statistical Association. Ethical guidelines for statistical practice: executive Summary. *Amstat News*. April 1999:12–15.
4. Lenth RV. Some practical guidelines for effective sample size determination. *Am Stat*. 2001;55:187–193.
5. Toto RD, Adams-Huet B, Fenves AZ, et al. Effect of ramipril on blood pressure and protein excretion rate in normotensive nondiabetic patients with proteinuria. *Am J Kidney Dis*. 1996;28:832–840.
6. Dupont WD, Plummer WD, Jr. Power and sample size calculations. A review and computer program. *Control Clin Trials*. 1990;11:116–128. Available at: http://biostat.mc.vanderbilt.edu/twiki/bin/view/Main/PowerSampleSize
7. Ahn C, Jung SH. Effect of dropouts on sample size estimates for test on trends across repeated measurements. *J Biopharm Stat*. 2005;15:33–41.
8. Ahn C. Sample size requirement for clinical trials with repeated binary outcomes. *Drug Inf J*. 2008;42:107–113.
9. Lancaster GA, Dodd S, Williamson PR. Design and analysis of pilot studies: recommendations for good practice. *J Eval Clin Pract*. 2004;10:307–312.
10. Pocock S. *Clinical Trials: A Practical Approach*. New York: John Wiley and Sons; 1983.
11. Day SJ, Altman DG. Statistics notes: blinding in clinical trials and other studies. *BMJ*. 2000;321:504.
12. International Conference on Harmonisation (ICH). Guidance for industry: E9 statistical principles for clinical trials. Rockville, MD: Food and Drug Administration; September 1998.
13. Friedman LM, CD Furberg, DeMets DL. *Fundamentals of Clinical Trials*. 3rd ed. New York: Springer; 1998.
14. Lachin JM. Statistical considerations in the intent-to-treat principle. *Control Clin Trials*. 2000;21:167–189.
15. Altman D. *Practical Statistics for Medical Research*. New York: Chapman and Hall/CRC; 1991.
16. Chow S-C, Jen-Pei L. *Design and Analysis of Clinical Trials: Concepts and Methodologies*. New York: John Wiley and Sons; 1998.
17. Rossouw JE, Anderson GL, Prentice RL, et al. Risks and benefits of estrogen plus progestin in healthy postmenopausal women: principal results from the Women's Health Initiative randomized controlled trial. *JAMA*. 2002;288:321–333.
18. Pocock SJ. Group sequential methods in the design and analysis of clinical trials. *Biometrika*. 1977;64:191–200.
19. O'Brien PC, Fleming TR. A multiple testing procedure for clinical trials. *Biometrics*. 1979; 35:549–556.
20. DeMets DL, Lan KK. Interim analysis: the alpha spending function approach. *Stat Med*. 1994;13:1341–1352; discussion 53–56.
21. Daya S. Strategies to control confounding in causation studies. *Evidence-based Obstet Gynecol*. 2002;4:1–2.

CHAPTER 6

Protocol Implementation Procedures

Tammy L. Lightfoot, RN, BSN

INTRODUCTION

A clinical trial protocol is a diagram of the entire study that provides a detailed explanation of the purpose of the study, background information about the disease or condition, study design, inclusion and exclusion criterion, procedures and treatments (investigational product [IP] or device), and the methodology that will be used to analyze the data collected. The study protocol is the guide that the investigator and the study staff follow to ensure that the study procedures are followed to maintain the study integrity, reduce errors, and protect the safety of the participants.

A study protocol may be developed by an investigator (investigator initiated) for a single site with funding from the National Institutes of Health (NIH), a pharmaceutical company, or other private funding sources. Multicenter protocols are most often funded by the NIH or a pharmaceutical company. Typically multicenter trials solicited by the NIH are developed by a consortium of investigators from different sites in collaboration with NIH officials. In this case the protocol is prepared by the consortium and approved by the NIH to ensure that it meets the goals of the NIH sponsor. Pharmaceutical industry-sponsored clinical trials follow a similar process in which the sponsor invites experienced scientists to assist them in developing and implementing the study protocol for a multicenter study.

PROTOCOL IMPLEMENTATION PREPARATION

Whether a protocol is developed by the investigator or sponsor, the investigator must be prepared to implement the protocol first by completing the following tasks:

- Acquiring funding
- Gathering study-specific resources
- Staff training
- Regulatory approval (institutional approval and other regulatory agencies, if applicable) of the protocol and all relevant documents

FUNDING

During the study design phase an investigator should start identifying funding sources. If the protocol is developed based on a response to an NIH funding opportunity announcement (FOA), the investigator should carefully read the announcement instructions and be aware of the submission deadline and the limitations on the actual amount of funding allowed. For additional details on preparing a budget see Chapter 10.

Adequate funding is critical to the successful completion of a clinical trial; therefore, careful and thoughtful development of a study budget tailored to the scientific protocol is essential. Inadequate funding can result in an inability to properly conduct a clinical trial. Funding shortfalls can result in midstream changes to the protocol such as deletion of diagnostic tests and procedures or worse, early termination of the study and inconclusive results.

For industry-sponsored trials, the investigator's budget is based on a negotiated budget/contract agreement between the investigator and the sponsor. However, whether a clinical trial is funded by the investigator, the NIH, or a pharmaceutical company, the investigator must ensure that he or she has the appropriate funding to start and finish the clinical trial. For example, if the investigator is conducting a trial in a facility that requires overhead costs to be subtracted from the budget (indirect cost), the investigator must plan to conduct the study based on the amount left after the overhead is subtracted (direct costs). Therefore, an investigator must know the percentage rate of the indirect costs at his or her institution when planning the protocol budget for the type of grant or

RESEARCH ETHICS: PITFALLS & PRESCRIPTIONS

Funding needs can lurk in unexpected places, with substantive ethical implications. For instance, consider normal-control studies involving imaging or genome scanning. Does your study have funding for reading/interpreting abnormal, clinically significant, unexpected findings?

Illes J, Kirschen MP, Edwards E, et al. Views & reviews: practical approaches to incidental findings in brain imaging research. *Neurology*. 2008;70:384–390.

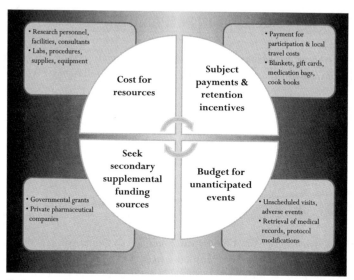

FIGURE **6-1**   Protocol funding tips. It illustrates the major funding issues that should be considered during the study design phase to ensure sufficient funding for the allocation of resources.

contract that is being sought. With this in mind, the investigator might consider searching for additional funding from other sources (private or government) to supplement the primary budget to ensure adequate funding to support the resources needed for the clinical trial **(Figure 6-1)**.

RESOURCES

The resources needed to implement a protocol may vary based on the disease or condition, if a drug or device is involved, and the type of tests and procedures performed. Therefore, the investigator must research what is needed during the study design phase, in order to determine what resources are available, how they will utilize the resources, and how they will gain access to the resources that they do not have that are necessary to conduct the clinical trial. This type of information will help the investigator plan to develop a budget to allocate funding for the following study-specific resources:

- Coinvestigators
- Study staff (e.g., study coordinators and biostatistician)
- Space
- Equipment (e.g., diagnostic devices and computers) cost
- Supplies (medical and administrative)
- Recruitment and retention strategies
- Travel costs (investigator meetings, local travel to off campus sites)
- The cost to outsource services (e.g., study coordinator, diagnostic procedures, inpatient research admission, etc.)
- Participants' stipends and incentives

Searching for resources later may cause delays in starting the study and missed opportunities to recruit potential participants, which could result in the investigator's failure to meet the enrollment goal.

STAFF TRAINING

Protocol training must take place before the protocol is implemented. The NIH, the sponsor, or the investigator may conduct protocol training. The type of study (observational, interventional, drug or device, etc.) will determine the type of training that is required. Protocol training requirements vary based on the protocol procedures. Below is a basic list of training activities that will apply to most clinical trials:

- Protocol and consent review
- Standard Operating Procedures (SOP): standardization of procedures in a facility to enhance staff performance and consistency
- Manual of Operations: how to perform the procedures
- Health Insurance Portability and Accountability Act (HIPAA): a federal law passed by the Department of Health and Human Services to protect patients' medical information and access to their medical information
- Human Subjects Training: a review of guidelines and federal laws that protects the rights of human subjects in clinical trial
- Good Clinical Practice (GCP): a standard of practice that an investigator, the research staff, the study monitors, and the sponsors follow to ensure participant safety and integrity of the study
- The collection and processing of biological samples
- International Air Transport Association (IATA): training to properly and safely ship biologic specimens according to federal guidelines

Whether protocol training is conducted by the NIH, the investigator, or a pharmaceutical company, it is ultimately the investigator's responsibility to ensure that the research staff has undergone training to execute the protocol procedures. A well-designed clinical trial training program will accomplish the following results:

- Increase participant safety
- Minimize study errors
- Conduct study procedures and test as defined by the protocol
- Reduce the number of protocol deviations
- Safeguard integrity of the study
- Enhance the research staff knowledge and skills to deliver care and educate the study participants about the study procedures

REGULATORY APPROVAL

Under FDA regulations, an institutional review board (IRB) is an appropriately constituted group that has been formally designated to review and monitor biomedical research involving human subjects. In accordance with FDA regulations, an IRB has the authority to approve, require modifications (to secure approval), or not approve a clinical trial protocol. The purpose of the IRB is to assure, both in advance and by periodic annual reviews, that the appropriate steps are taken to protect the rights and welfare of humans participating in clinical trials. To accomplish this purpose, IRBs use a group process (scientific and laypeople who are not involved with the clinical trial) to review research protocols and related materials (e.g., informed consent, investigator brochures, recruitment and retention material, and participants' stipends and incentives) (see Chapters 2 and 3).

THE INVESTIGATOR'S RESPONSIBILITIES

The investigator may delegate the responsibility to a designee (study coordinator, fellow, or administrator) to prepare and submit the protocol, the consent form (if applicable), and all other relevant documents; however, the investigator is responsible for ensuring that the IRB has all the information for the review process. Failure to submit the appropriate documents and respond to the IRB review questions (stipulations) will result in protocol implementation delays. Therefore, the investigator must be prepared to respond quickly to the IRB's stipulations. This may require the investigator or designee to present to the changes requested by the IRB to the sponsor to ensure that they agree with the changes before final IRB approval. Failure to communicate the IRB stipulations to the sponsor will result in protocol implementation delays and loss of funding if the sponsor will not agree to the changes.

SUMMARY

The medical community and public health rely on results from evidence-based clinical trials to set the standard for the medical management of patients. The successful implementation of a clinical trial protocol will bring investigators a step closure to discovering new drugs and treatments that will change the course of health care and improve quality of life globally. Investigators are charged with the responsibility to serve communities by developing and implementing protocols that will capture, measure, and translate research data into meaningful information that can be used by health care providers to deliver effective and high-quality health care. Therefore, the investigator must meticulously gather information to develop a sufficient budget to ensure that the appropriate resources are acquired and staff training is completed to execute a clinical trial protocol.

CHAPTER 7

Screening and Evaluation

Robert D. Toto, MD

OUTLINE

Introduction	Special Tests
Infrastructure	Screen Failures
Identify clinic space needs	Documentation
Advertising	Study visit and documentation
Operations	Source documentation
Time allocation	Customizing case report forms
Screening and Evaluation Visit: 10 Steps	Screening and Evaluation Study Forms
Protocol-Specific Requirements	

INTRODUCTION

The recruitment and retention of study subjects is the key to the success of any form of clinical and translational research project. In order to efficiently and effectively recruit study subjects who are willing and able, to participate in a study, it is first necessary to put in place the appropriate infrastructure, operations, and documentation to optimize screening and evaluation. This chapter discusses screening and evaluation methods and techniques applicable to any patient-oriented research project.

INFRASTRUCTURE

Identify Clinic Space Needs

Clinic space location is important should ideally be made as convenient as possible for potential study subjects. This is not always possible to control by the investigator but should be a priority for location for junior investigators. It is always preferable to conduct screening on site of the investigators' laboratory or office, but screening at off-site locations may be needed in some circumstances in order to achieve recruitment goal. Investigators should estimate the amount of space needed to conduct the screening and evaluation process then set about identifying the space and equipping it accordingly.

The space must be secure to protect confidential information whether written or stored in encrypted computer data files.

A minimum amount of space should include an interview and examination room for the study subject and office space for the individual(s) who will conduct the screening and evaluation process. Two hundred square feet of properly equipped space can be effective and efficient for conducting several studies simultaneously depending on the size of the study populations and protocol specifics. The space should include desktop and file cabinet, telephone, fax, copy machine, and at least one computer with Internet connection. A typical outpatient examination room with an examination table, height and weight station, desktop, storage for patient examination and study supplies, measuring devices (e.g., sphygmomanometer, scale, etc.), sink for hand washing, and blood sampling supplies should also be within the clinic space. A refrigerator with a $-20°C$ freezer and tabletop centrifuge for preparing body fluid samples is recommended for collection of blood and body fluid at screening or evaluation visits. The office space should include supplies for documentation and for creating labels and preparing samples for shipping and receiving as needed. It is highly desirable to have private bathroom within the research space, but a separate private bathroom facility nearby research clinic enclosure is workable.

The office space should be large enough for the investigator to conduct brief meetings with research team members (e.g., research nurse, collaborators). The examination room and office space should be separated from one another when possible so that privacy is ensured. In case screening and evaluation procedures must take place in the hospital setting, the patient's hospital room and doctor's station may suffice. In this setting the investigator must be able to carry informed consent forms and data collection forms (or a laptop computer for data collection). Investigators should design and arrange screening and evaluation clinic space in a manner that allows for security of study documents.

ADVERTISING

A variety of methods for advertising for studies are available to investigators including written materials for posting and mailing as well as Internet sites, newspapers, or other written materials. The success of these methods is highly dependent on the location and specifics of the study and should be tailored accordingly. Whatever method(s) is used, they must receive prior institutional review board (IRB) approval and in some cases approval by the study sponsor. Mass mailings are more effective if they are followed up by phone contact. Partnering with health care organizations for advertising studies that require large numbers of study subjects is another helpful method assisting in the recruitment of screenees. These methods are described in greater detail in other chapters (see Chapters 2, 8, and 12).

OPERATIONS

Time Allocation

It is critically important for the investigator to estimate amount of time needed to conduct a screening interview, obtain informed consent, perform screening tests (e.g., blood, etc.), and perform evaluations. These may include medical history, physical examination, and measurements prior to implementing the first study subject visit. For example, screening tests may include blood pressure, mental health questionnaires, or other key data needed for study eligibility.

Another key aspect of screening and evaluation is to estimate the number of screening visits needed to achieve the recruitment goal for a given study. In order to enroll a subject in a study, one must screen and evaluate the patient first. By accurately estimating the ratio of screenees to enrollees the investigator can more efficiently enroll study subjects, a prerequisite to successfully completing a research project within the time specified by the study protocol. A good way to go about this is to interview successful investigators who have conducted similar studies as the ratio of screenee to enrolled study subject may vary considerably from study to study. An accurate estimate of the screening to enrollment ratio provides a measure of efficiency of the conduct of study and is useful for computing the time needed to conduct future studies. In addition, calculating the time it takes to conduct a screening visit allows the investigator to determine how many screening visits can be conducted on a daily/weekly basis. This information should be tracked and entered into a database for inclusion in preliminary data sections of future grant applications and IRB protocols.

When conducting screening visits, it is advisable, whenever possible, to offer a flexible schedule for study subjects in order to enhance enrollment. Providing potential candidates with information (preferably in writing) on location, hours of operation, what to expect at the screening visit, and the length of the visit is important. Depending on the location of the clinic, it may be advisable to provide an escort for the study subject to locate the clinic to facilitate their on-time arrival. Compliance with the Health Insurance Portability and Accountability Act (HIPPA) as well as IRB principles and guidelines is an important part of the screening process. Documentation of provision of HIPAA and IRB documents to potential study subjects is an important part of the screening process. For details on procurement and use of these instruments see Chapters 8 and 12 on subject recruitment and data collection.

SCREENING AND EVALUATION VISIT: 10 STEPS

The purpose of the screening visit is to begin the process for confirming eligibility, meeting potential study subjects, obtaining informed consent, and collecting necessary data to proceed toward enrollment. The screening and evaluation visit can be broken down into 10 key steps **(Table 7-1)**.

Step 1: Educate the study subject (and family members, if permitted) the purpose of the research and why the study subject is considered a potential candidate for the research. The concept that the study subject is part of the research team should be introduced to the study subject and emphasized. Obviously, patient-oriented research cannot be conducted without study subjects; therefore, it is vital to convey this concept to potential study subjects.

Step 2: Provide study subject with a copy of the IRB approved, written informed consent form and permitted time to read it thoroughly. It is important to be sure that the study subject thoroughly understands the informed consent. Often study subjects may wish to take the consent form home and review it with family members.

TABLE **7-1** | Ten Steps for Screening and Evaluating Potential
Study Subjects

Step	Purpose
1. Obtain informed consent	Allow next steps to take place
2. Educate study subject	Engage and inform subject about the importance of the project and their participation
3. Answer questions	Build relationship with subject
4. Collect eligibility data	Phenotype the study subject (inclusion and exclusion criteria)
5. Provide written instructions	Ensure understanding of procedures and follow up
6. Document findings	Accountability and capture of critical study data
7. Principal investigator review	Ensure that subject is an appropriate candidate
8. Inclusion and exclusion criteria checklist	Ensure integrity of the study sample and prevent protocol violation
9. Document on case report form	Ensure accuracy and integrity of the study data
10. Enroll study subject	Allow next steps/procedures for study to proceed

Step 3: Invite and answer questions. The study subject and family members should be invited to ask questions and the person obtaining consent should provide answers to the best of their ability. If the investigator or study personnel obtaining consent cannot answer a question immediately, it should be written down, the answer should be researched and provided to the potential study subject as soon as possible. Providing answers builds credibility even if the subject does not decide to participate or is found to be ineligible. The study subject will appreciate your efforts and may be more likely to accept an invitation to participate in a future study. The study subject should sign and date the consent form indicating that they have read it and understand the study (for details about the composition see Chapter 3 on informed consent).

Step 4: Collect eligibility data including medical history, physical examination/vital signs questionnaires, and laboratory/other tests needed to confirm eligibility (see inclusion and exclusion criteria). During this time, potential subjects may be given verbal instruction about details of the study covered in the consent form or in additional written materials to be provided at a later date.

Step 5: Provide verbal and written instructions to the potential study subject for the next communication or enrollment visit. This step is important since study subjects not previously involved in research often need reassurance that they are part of the study team and in fact the most important part.

Step 6: Document the above steps on study-specific data collection forms. A signed copy of the informed written consent should be provided to the study subject and kept on file in the investigator's office. Importantly, it cannot be overemphasized that appropriate

RESEARCH ETHICS: PITFALLS & PRESCRIPTIONS

Much of the time, the ability of a potential research participant to understand and consent to a protocol is taken for granted. However, in the case of some subject populations the ability to understand and consent to the research may be limited (children, some mentally ill individuals, or cognitively impaired individuals). In these cases, special federal regulations apply and may require either an assessment of the individual's ability to consent, a proxy decision maker or study companion, or special consideration by the IRB. Prisoners and probationers also require special consideration because of perceived or actual constraints on voluntary participation in this population. Research with individuals involved in criminal conduct (typically, substance abuse) may also require special precautions because of the ethics of protecting privacy, as well as the pragmatic consideration of enabling populations to feel safe to participate. All these ethical and regulatory considerations should be addressed before the investigator is actually engaged in recruitment.

Miller FG. Recruiting research participants. In: Emanuel E, Grady C, Crouch RA, et al., eds. *The Oxford Textbook of Clinical Research Ethics.* New York: Oxford University Press; 2008:397–403.

documentation of study subject information is recorded and securely stored for future reference (for more details see Chapter 12 on data collection).

Step 7: Review by the principal investigator of the screening and eligibility data. This step is done to ensure that the study subject is eligible for further evaluation and subsequent enrollment in the study.

Step 8: Review the inclusion and exclusion criteria checklist. This step is designed to ensure that the study subject meets all the criteria specified in the protocol. A checklist including all inclusion and exclusion criteria should be created and customized prior to the first study subject screening visit and employed at this step (see below under Source Documentation).

Step 9: Document the review of the screening and evaluation and inclusion and exclusion criteria. This step is designed to ensure accuracy and integrity of the study data.

Step 10: Enroll eligible study subject and proceed with the study protocol. The study subject should be reminded of the next steps and provided written instructions for next study procedure / visit.

PROTOCOL-SPECIFIC REQUIREMENTS

Providing written instructions for subsequent visits is the final step after the screening and evaluation visit. The instructions must include when the next contact will take place, the method (e.g., telephone, revisit), when it is planned, and the location. If the location differs from the location of the screening and evaluation visit, directions and telephone contacts should be provided to the potential study subject. This information must also be documented. In addition, if reimbursement for travel, time for study visits, or procedures are provided as noted in the consent form and process, it is advisable to remind the study subject of such provisions. Study team members who make contact with the potential study subject during the visit need to thank the potential study subject for taking the time to undergo screening and evaluation.

SPECIAL TESTS

In some instances, study-specific and prespecified requirements may involve collaborations with other investigators. These should be explained to the study subject and also when appropriate samples will be collected. For example, collection and storage of tissue samples and conducting special laboratory and imaging tests may be part of this process. Preparations for carrying out these procedures should be in place prior to the screening visit. For example, special storage receptacles for tissue, special tubes or conditions for blood collection and imaging equipment, and requisite technical skills to make measurements should be available and convenient for potential study subjects.

SCREEN FAILURES

Inevitably, some potential study subjects will fail to pass the screening criteria, also known as screen failures. A "screen failure" is defined as a study subject who does not meet the inclusion and exclusion criteria for the study. There are several important reasons to document and catalog the reasons for screen failures in any given study. First, it provides important information regarding the feasibility of recruiting study subjects from your site. Second, some study protocols permit rescreening of potential study subjects after a designated time interval. Third, protocol modifications may be justified and implemented based on frequency of screen failures when the reason for screen failures is common among the study population of interest.

Hypothetical example 1: An investigator needs one additional study subject to complete enrollment, and a screenee meets all inclusion criteria except for the exclusion criteria of a body mass index (BMI) of 45 kg/m². However, the current screenee has a BMI of 46 kg/m². This subject has by definition failed screening by not meeting all of the exclusion criteria. The question is: Now what do you do? In this case, the investigator should by protocol exclude this potential participant. Still, one might ask whether it is appropriate to request the subject to lose enough weight to meet this criterion. Another question is whether the investigator should make an exception and enroll the subject and document the reason for the exception. In this circumstance the investigator should exclude the subject from further evaluation. However, this example brings up the issue of rescreening study subjects who do not meet all inclusion and exclusion criteria. Rescreening the above subject may be permitted if prespecified in the written IRB-approved protocol. Alternatively, during the screening for the study, an investigator may modify an existing protocol and request a protocol amendment be approved by the appropriate IRB. In some studies, for example a multicenter study, the study sponsor must also approve protocol amendments.

Hypothetical example 2: A potential study subject on blood pressure medication is screened for a blood pressure study in which the screening systolic blood pressure must be ≥130 mm Hg. However, at the visit the subject is found to have a SBP of 128 mm Hg. In this case, the study protocol was prespecified for this occurrence and was approved by the IRB. Specifically, a second (optional) screening visit was built into the study protocol. Specifically, the IRB-approved protocol stipulated that "if systolic blood pressure level during screening visit is below 130 mmHg for subjects on antihypertensive therapy, a second screening visit may be conducted to repeat systolic blood pressure for eligibility and entry into the study. Potential subjects are advised to return within 1–2 weeks for this second visit. In addition, medication back titration may be performed at the discretion of the principal investigator to achieve the inclusion goal and to avoid a precipitous rise in blood pressure. If SBP remains <130 mm Hg the potential participant is excluded." Note that in this example, specifics for rescreening for this particular enrollment criterion such as the time interval, the role of the principal investigator, and the outcome of the second visit are specified. Building in rescreening may be useful to assist in study subject recruitment in certain circumstances and should be considered in the planning stages for the study.

These examples illustrate that flexibility in study procedures can be built into study protocols or be achieved by protocol amendments provided they are approved by the IRB and, when appropriate, the study sponsor.

DOCUMENTATION

Study Visit and Documentation

Study subject procedures should be protocol driven. The process for the screening evaluation should specify the rationale for a screening visit, the function of the visit, the amount of time it is estimated to take to conduct a screening visit, under what conditions and where the visit will take place, and who will conduct the screening visit. The details including the time and timing of the visit should be specified in the protocol and followed during the visit. In addition, the sources of information used in the clinic visit should be specified and documented during the visit. For example, how the study subject was contacted for the screening visit, what information was available to the research team to identify the potential study subject, and documentation of this information should be performed at this visit.

Source Documentation

Documenting the source of information collected at the screening visit is essential. In most instances the information is collected directly from the study subject; however, family members may also provide information on the medical history or other aspects for the study subject's lifestyle that may be important in the screening process. Information may also be obtained from a paper- or computer-based medical record and these sources may vary from subject to subject. Information from the referring physician of the subject may also be available and prove valuable in determining eligibility for the study. Documentation of data collected at the study visit is important for both regulatory purposes and for investigator use in the current and future studies. Study-specific case report forms for the screening procedure should be created and utilized for each potential study subjects (see Chapter 9 for examples). These forms may be in paper form or may be computer based and should be filled out at the time of the screening visit. The data should ideally be put into an encrypted computer database that is backed up by a secure external media source (e.g., external hard drive, server, etc.).

Customizing Case Report Forms

Generic forms for collection of medical history and examination may be used for many studies; nevertheless, the amount of medical information needed is often study specific. For example, some studies require limited and others complete information on medical history and examination. Whenever possible, concordance between the written medical history and the study subject's medical history should be obtained. For example, obtaining medical records that document a history of a myocardial infarction can be important particularly in studies of cardiovascular disease. Obtaining medical records from the study subject or their physician's office and hospital records may be necessary to confirm components of the medical history depending on the specifics of the inclusion and exclusion criteria of your study. In cases where a family member is present and with permission of the study subject, supplemental or corroborative information on medical history may be procured. If a physical examination is required during the screening and evaluation visit, protocol specifics should be followed and the findings should be recorded. If incidental physical finding abnormalities are noted, for example an unexpected cutaneous lesion or an abdominal mass, the study subject should be notified and after the visit is completed this information should be transmitted to the subject's primary care physician. Such findings may or may not result in exclusion from the study, but it is important to bring them to the attention of subject and physician and to document the transmission of this information to both.

Screening and Evaluation Study Forms

Study-specific forms facilitate data collection, documentation, and future data retrieval, and should be labeled with the study title and number (if applicable). These forms should include inclusion and exclusion criteria, key information on eligibility, subject demographics, and other data as needed. The inclusion and exclusion criteria should be identical to those in the written protocol and should be listed on the form in a checklist format. Key information on eligibility may be included on a study-specific medical history form. Subject demographics and other data such as the subject's primary care physician or special medical information should be collected. The "other" information is very important for future use in the event that the subject screens in and is enrolled into the study.

All screening documents as well as other documents used in the study should be identified by document type and include date and time. A hard copy of these documents should be kept in secured locations in a study binder and/or in a computer database. A screening study log should be utilized to list those who have completed a screening visit and at minimum the date and time of screening, name of study subject, and disposition (e.g., screened in/screen failure). This log provides a rapid way for the investigators to determine the screen failure rate and the reason(s) for screen failure. A checklist of study procedures carried out at the screening visit should be completed by study personnel and stored in the study database. The checklist includes the following:

- Consent(s)/HIPAA(s) are IRB approved with current approval/expiration dates.
- Consent(s)/HIPAA(s) are read by participant.
- Consent(s)/HIPAA(s) are read to participant by study staff.
- Purpose, duration, procedures, and possible risks were fully explained to the participant.
- The participant's questions/concerns were answered by the study staff (see Screening and Evaluation Visit and Table 7.1).
- Participant acknowledges their understanding and willingness to participate in this research study by date and signature.
- Copy of signed and dated consent(s)/HIPAA(s) is given to participant.
- Original signed and dated consent(s)/HIPAA(s) are placed in participant's research chart.
- These informed consent(s)/HIPAA(s) were signed by the participant prior to any study-related procedures in our research clinic.

CHAPTER 8

Recruitment and Retention

Tammy L. Lightfoot, RN, BSN

INTRODUCTION

The recruitment and retention of study participants are vital for the successful completion of any clinical trial. In today's research climate a broad range of resources, from sophisticated multimedia advertising campaigns, global call centers serving multiple sites, Internet postings, and direct mailings can all be called into play to supplement traditional methods to identify and connect with potential participants. The advent of the Health Insurance Portability and Accountability Act (HIPAA), which protects a patient's privacy and access to their health information, has had an important impact on the common practices of record review and use of databases thereby engendering alternative approaches to recruitment necessary.

An investigator may have a well-designed trial that is cognizant of the potential variables and utilizes the appropriate analytical methods to reduce outcome bias; however, if the appropriate number of participants are not recruited and retained the statistical power of the study to test the scientific hypothesis may be jeopardized. Therefore, a researcher must be proactive and creative in developing strategies that will circumvent recruitment and retention barriers. The primary goal of the information provided is intended to serve as a foundation or a blueprint for investigators to develop strategies that are unique to their clinical trial.

WHEN SHOULD RECRUITMENT AND RETENTION START?

An investigator should start strategizing recruitment and retention efforts during the study design phase. The study design phase is the time when the researcher is collecting data relating to how he or she will answer the study hypothesis. During this time, the researcher should start thinking about how to gain access to the target population, the types of analytical and diagnostic measurements, and resources that will be required to answer the study hypothesis. By addressing these questions early during the study design phase, the researcher will have the opportunity to identify potential barriers that could potentially impede the recruitment and retention of study participants. After a study protocol has undergone final approval by an Institutional Review Board (IRB) and obtained other required regulatory approvals, the investigator is ready to implement recruitment and retention strategies.

What are Recruitment and Retention Strategies?

Recruitment and retention strategies are tools developed that are study and participant specific to encourage and promote study compliance from the investigator, study team, and the participants. Investigators must first understand what the potential barriers are for the targeted population to develop effective methodologies to implement strategies that will reduce the impact of specific barriers identified from researching the characteristics of the target population. This approach will also reduce the cost by obviating ineffective strategies. Recruitment and retention tools will be discussed later in this chapter.

The Who, What, and How (WWH) Strategy

The WWH Strategy is a pragmatic approach for the development of study-specific recruitment and retention strategies to enhance a researcher's ability to complete a clinical trial. The application of the WWH Strategy to the six components below will help the investigator select the appropriate approaches to move forward with the implementation of a clinical trial:

1. The disease or condition
2. Inclusion and exclusion criteria
3. Study procedures
4. Duration of study
5. Funding
6. Resources

The Disease or Condition

The disease or condition the investigator is studying will define WHO will be the study population. The study population will determine WHAT sites to utilize for recruitment and if the sample size can be supported from the proposed recruitment sites. An investigator should also consider participant characteristics like age, gender, social and economical status, culture, ethnicity, educational level, literacy, and vulnerability (e.g., prisoners, children, and the elderly). The prevalence of the disease may also influence the investigator's ability to recruit enough participants to statistically power the study. These are all important variables that could pose potential barriers hindering recruitment and retention efforts. Therefore, the investigator should consider HOW he or she might develop realistic strategies to reduce the negative impact of these variables on recruitment and retention.

Inclusion and Exclusion Criteria

The inclusion and exclusion criteria are designed to ensure the enrollment of the appropriate study participants to determine if the treatment (drug or device) is effective and safe for the intended patient population. However, overly stringent inclusion and exclusion criteria can lead to low enrollment and revisions resulting in costly study extensions and delays. Therefore, a researcher should research WHO has conducted clinical trials associated with the disease they are studying, WHAT type of study design was used, and the results of those trials. This information will allow the researcher determine HOW to construct a feasible study design, and inclusion and exclusion criteria to ensure enrollment of the appropriate study participants and maximize the likelihood of achieving the recruitment goal.

Study Procedures

During the study design phase, the investigator must decide which procedures are truly required to test the study hypothesis. Complicated study procedures can negatively influence participant recruitment and retention. In some instances, participants are reluctant to enroll in a clinical trial if the procedures are too invasive, painful, time consuming, and inconvenient. The protocol background and rationale sections are the primary sections that will guide the investigator in the right direction regarding WHAT procedures are needed, and WHO and HOW will the procedures be conducted to answer the study hypothesis. Focusing on those procedures that are necessary for completing the study and avoiding excessive, invasive, and time-consuming procedures that are not focused on the main research question will facilitate both recruitment and retention.

Study Duration

The duration of a clinical trial could also influence a participant's decision to enroll and remain in a trial. The retention of participants in long-term trials is difficult. For example, during long-terms trials, participants are more likely to become lost to follow-up due to relocation, transportation and family issues, coexisting medical illnesses, and a loss of interest and death. One method commonly used to adjust for participant loss is to over-recruit participants. During the study design this over-recruitment is generally built into the recruitment goal after discussion with the biostatistician. The exact number of participants needed for statistical power is determined by an estimate to include the number of subjects who may not complete the study. For example, in a study that needs 100 subjects to test the hypothesis, it is incumbent on the investigator to estimate a "drop out" rate. In this example if a 10% drop out rate is estimated then the number is $100/(1 - 0.1) = 111$ subjects. Over-recruitment can provide additional security that the researcher will have enough completers for data analysis. If this approach is used, the investigator should inform the IRB of the intended number of participants needed to reach the randomization goal during the initial IRB review submission to avoid submitting a modification to the IRB that could delay recruitment efforts. For example, if 20 participants were needed to power the study, the investigator might inform the IRB that 40 participants might be recruited to reach the randomization goal if a 50% drop out rate during the screening and evaluation period is anticipated. Once the investigator researches the randomization goal of 20, recruitment would end.

In some cases, the investigator must employ complicated clinical measurements and require long-term participation to statistically validate the clinical trial results. However, whether a trial is short term or long term, the investigator should pre-plan for potential problems during the study design phase by considering WHO the participants are. WHAT frequency of follow-up visits and procedures are required, where they will take place, and HOW will they acquire the appropriate level of resources and funding needed to ensure that the appropriate procedures and tests are funded to answer the study hypothesis.

Application of the WWH Rule for Multicenter Clinical Trials

The WWH strategy can also apply to multicenter industry-sponsored trials. Before contract negotiations are started, the sponsor will complete their selection process to determine if the investigator has the appropriate experience, staff, participant population, and resources to conduct their clinical trial. During the site selection process, the sponsor will ask specific questions to determine WHO the investigator's population is, WHAT resources the investigator has to conduct the clinical trial (e.g., facility, staff, laboratory, and equipment), and HOW the participants will be recruited and retained. Today, due to the competitive atmosphere among the pharmaceutical and device industry to get their product on the market, many sponsors are providing recruitment and retention tools to help clinical sites meet their recruitment and retention goals.

Funding

Inadequate funding will affect the investigator's ability to properly conduct a clinical trial. Understanding WHO your participant population is, WHAT is needed to gain access to potential recruitment sites, and HOW to logistically recruit and retain participants will all influence the clinical trial cost.

For investigator-initiated trials, the investigator usually obtains funding from federal and industry sources to support their research endeavors. In some cases, funding cannot be obtained until there is a completed IRB-approved protocol; however, the investigator must be proactive in identifying funding sources early during the study design phase to avoid delays initiating their trial due to lack of funding.

Resources

Resources are one of the most important components a researcher must have to conduct a clinical trial to ensure that the study is completed and the integrity of the data is protected.

The type of resources needed by an investigator is defined by the protocol design. Below is a simple list of the basic resources needed for a clinical trial:

1. Research team
2. Space
3. Training
4. Supplies for diagnostic specimens and shipping supplies
5. Access to diagnostic services (if needed)

Know what your resources are and where to find the resources you do not have! Searching for resources later may cause

1. Start-up delays
2. Missing potential subjects for recruitment
3. Failure to meet recruitment goals
4. Inability to complete the study

Resource Networking

If an investigator is new or has limited resources, networking with other well-established investigators as coinvestigators or collaborators might lead to access to invaluable resources (e.g., space, trained staff, and laboratory) to conduct a clinical trail. In addition, sharing resources like a study coordinator, space, supplies, and costly diagnostic services is a cost-effective approach to reduce study costs. However, if the trial is a multicenter industry-sponsored trial, the sponsor will usually provide the study supplies, centralized laboratory and protocol training, but it is the investigator's responsibility to ensure adequate, safe, and accessible space for the participants.

BUILDING A CLINICAL RESEARCH TEAM

The investigator must invest in building a research team that consists of individuals (e.g., study coordinator, coinvestigators, biostatistician, research and laboratory technicians, and administrative support) that have the level of expertise required to navigate through the various study challenges. The protocol specifics will determine the type of personnel and training required to safely and efficiently carryout the protocol procedures. However, budget constraints can be challenging particularly with regard to an investigator's ability to hire and retain trained personnel. To reduce personnel cost, the investigator must identify individuals that are knowledgeable about clinical trials and can multitask. A study coordinator is usually the person that can fulfill this description. Although the investigator is responsible for the clinical trial conduct, the study coordinator has a strong leadership role on clinical trials.

Training

A well-trained research team will enhance the investigator's ability to accomplish recruitment and retention goals. For multicentered trials, it is the sponsor's responsibility to ensure that the designated research staff completes study-specific training. However, for any trial, it is the investigator's responsibility to ensure that the research team has completed the sponsor's training, internal training that meets the Food and Drug Administration (FDA), the site's

IRB guidelines, and all other regulatory bodies to ensure the correct and safe delivery of care throughout the course of the study. Failure to train the research staff can result in participant injury, improperly collecting biological specimens, enrollment of participants not meeting the inclusion criteria, and poor and incomplete data collection. Ultimately, due to poor training or lack of training, the integrity of the trial and the investigator's reputation could be damaged, which could lead to the sponsor (federal or industry) withdrawing the study from the site and the funding. The different types of training are discussed in Chapter 6.

Study Coordinator

A study coordinator or clinical coordinator can make or break a clinical trial. The actual study procedures should determine if the study coordinator is a nurse or non-clinical individual. For example, in clinical trials with various medical procedures and assessments, a nurse may be more suitable as the study coordinator. A clinical trial limited to data collection may be more suitable for an unlicensed coordinator.

The study coordinator is a multifaceted individual that wears many hats **(Figure 8-1)**. Often, the study coordinator is responsible for completing the internal regulatory documents and submitting the study protocol to the IRB. Additionally, the study coordinator may perform the following study procedures: consenting participants, phlebotomy, referring participant for social services, participant advocate, capturing and entering participant data, and primary liaison to sponsor. Depending on the study population's social and economical

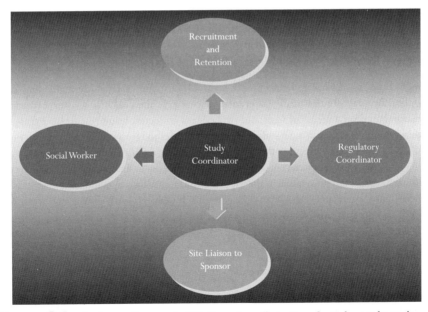

FIGURE **8-1**　Study coordinator role. This figure is an illustration of a study coordinator's skill diversity for a clinical trial. A coordinator must be prepared to serve many roles to facilitate recruitment and retention efforts. In many settings, the coordinator is at the center of the decision-making process because he or she has developed invaluable skills and relationships with the participant, sponsor, Institutional Review Board, and other key resource peoples that can be utilized to enhance recruitment and retention.

needs, the study coordinator may also assist study participants with finding social services to address their needs to promote retention. This individual is normally the first and last person to interact with participants, attend training meetings with the investigator, train new staff members, and develop and implement recruitment and retention strategies.

Consenting Process

Helping potential participants understand the distinction between research and standard care begins with the consenting process. This process is a dialogue between the personnel obtaining consent and the participant and their family (if applicable). The study staff designated to consent participants must have a clear understanding about the clinical trial purpose, procedures, duration, potential adverse events, and benefits (if applicable) to appropriately consent a participant. The consenting process is a voluntary process that must be completed prior to conducting any study procedure. The participant must be given ample time to read the consent and have all questions answered before signing the consent form. A standard consent should have the following key elements:

- What the study is about.
- Why the participant qualifies for screening and enrollment.
- Study procedures (lab tests, study drug, or device).
- What is expected of the participant and the length of their participation?
- What is considered experimental and standard of care in the study?
- What costs are the participant and investigator (or sponsor) responsible for?
- Treatment and responsibility for study-related injuries.

Differing Goals in Research Versus Standard Practice

In many cases, research and clinical practice activities are often carried out in the same setting, but the goals are drastically different. For research, the goal is to answer a research question based on a series of tests and procedures collected using research *participants* within a prescribed time using standardized scientific methods to validate the research findings. For a clinical practice, it is therapy. The goal is to provide medical treatment for an individual *patient* based on acceptable treatment protocols at a medical facility, or treatment that is generally acceptable in the medical community for a specific disease or illness. *Note:* Potential participants and their clinicians must be able to clearly grasp this distinction, since therapy may or may not occur with study participation.

Communication Cycle

A well-formed "Communication Cycle" **(Figure 8-2)** will facilitate the clear dissemination of information that will promote and enhance recruitment and retention. The study coordinator is usually the primary liaison between the key participants like the study participant, investigator, sponsor, and other individuals (e.g., the primary care provider (PCP), family members, and laboratory staff) that ensures ongoing communications throughout the course of the study. Communications should be circular allowing a continuous flow of information between the key participants. For example, if the PCP is not the investigator, the study coordinator is

RESEARCH ETHICS: PITFALLS & PRESCRIPTIONS

Communicating the difference between clinical trials and standard clinical care is difficult. Confusing the two—sometimes called the "therapeutic misconception"—is easy to do. The ethically crucial aspect is that the clinical research participant—by consenting to participate—gives up the privilege of tailored medical treatment to the individual's needs and preferences. Instead, the research participant agrees to the study procedures and research design, which narrow the participant's options. Three areas are particularly difficult for many subjects to understand—the control condition, the placebo, and randomization. Extra care is needed in explaining these concepts, and having the potential subject explain these aspects of study design to the investigator is a useful method for enhancing understanding.

Appelbaum P, Roth L, Lidz C, et al. False hopes and best data: consent to research and the therapeutic misconception. *Hastings Cent Rep.* 1987;17(2):20–24.

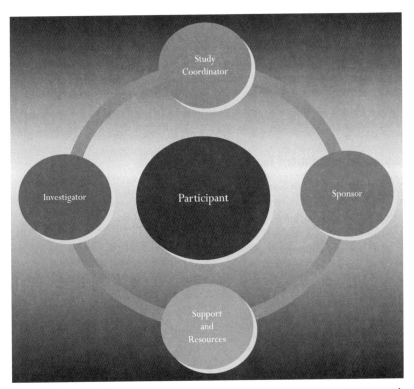

FIGURE **8-2**   Communication cycle. This figure shows a continuous communication cycle that is centered around the participant that includes all parties involved in the communication process to keep the participant informed and engaged during their participation in a clinical trial.

normally the first study team member to approach the PCP to request access to their patient population and provide updates to the PCP regarding the participants progress as instructed by the investigator to ensure continuity of care. The participant should be in the center of the communication cycle with the study team and other key participants creating a clear flow of information to keep all parties informed of information that is relevant to their participation.

Customer Service

Outstanding customer service should be demonstrated to participants at all times. The participants and referring/managing physicians should be respected as valued customers, study personnel trained in customer service techniques, the facility where the participants are seen should have a customer-friendly study environment, and the study staff should demonstrate appreciation to the participants for their contributions to the clinical trial. The development of study-specific recruitment and retention tools is a form of customer service to keep the participant engaged.

Note: Always say thank you to a participant at the end of each study visit. A simple thank you from the study staff is a simple and meaningful way of showing participant appreciation.

Recruitment and Retention Tools

Recruitment and retention tools can help identify, recruit, and retain study participants. These tools can also help the investigator to organize the logistics of a clinical trail. The investigator and the research staff should identify the most appropriate recruitment and retention tools that will be useful for the participants. For example, a recruitment booklet designed to explain in layman's terms the purpose of the study, what is required of the participants, and defining common research terms is a helpful educational tool, and it can make the consenting process easier for both the participant and the study staff.

Examples of Recruitment Tools

- Presentation of study during colleagues at luncheons, grand rounds, etc.
- Generic clinical trial participation information
- Study-specific brochure
- Study team contact information sheet
- Business card with study hotline number
- What to expect at each study visit
- FAQs about the study
- Personal study folder
- Provide transportation or restrict enrollment to participants within a reasonable distance
- Use of electronic medical records

Retention Tools

Retention tools should be designed to retain study participants and promote protocol adherence. These tools should be developed based on the study design and the participant needs. For example, an effective retention tool for participants enrolled in a study requiring study drugs (investigational product [IP]) could be a medication bag to store the IP versus a keychain. This simple tool will help the participant to keep track of their IP and serve as a reminder to take the IP, which could lead to better compliance.

Retention and adherence are distinct aspects of study conduct. They are both important and are typically conducted simultaneously in order to ensure that study goals are met and the integrity of the study is maintained.

Retention is keeping the participant enrolled.

Adherence is ensuring that the participant is in compliance with the study treatment and procedures.

Note: Poor retention and adherence will impact both the quality of study data and the study integrity.

Examples of Retention Tools

- Provide transportation
- Coffee, bottled water, snacks after fasting blood draws
- Evening and weekend clinic hours, flexible scheduling
- Incentive payments to acknowledge time commitment
- Offer ongoing participant/family education
- Study appointment calendar with visit window reminders
- Birthday and holiday cards

RESEARCH ETHICS: PITFALLS & PRESCRIPTIONS

Choosing the kind and monetary value of incentives is an investigator's art of balancing scientific interests and participants' interests. Too-generous incentives may exert undue influence and "buy" participation, while too-stingy incentives may undermine participation and unfairly burden the participant with unwanted personal expenses (travel, parking, missed work, etc.). Cash may be preferred, but is prone to loss and misuse (as in purchasing drugs of abuse in vulnerable populations), so many programs prefer gift cards suitable to the population (e.g., toy store cards for children). How beneficial (or not) the study procedure is to the participant also factors into the incentive equation.

Dickert N, Grady C. Incentives for research participants. In: Emanuel EJ, Grady C, Crouch RA, et al., ed. *The Oxford Textbook of Clinical Research Ethics.* New York: Oxford University Press; 2008:386–396.

- Medication and urine specimen carrying bags
- Study identification card with study staff contact information
- Appointment reminders (phone calls and reminders mailed)

Internal Recruitment and Retention Tools

Internal recruitment and retention tools are designed for the internal use by the investigator and research staff for the purpose of implementing and facilitating participant enrollment. In addition these tools facilitate staff compliance with the study protocol. The study sponsor or study staff should develop specific forms and data tracking methods to keep track of all study activities. For example, a referral form with a synopsis of the study, staff phone number, fax number, and inclusion and exclusion criteria can be distributed to medical providers who may be willing and able to identify and refer potential participants from their medical practice. Another useful tool is a study-specific electronic spreadsheet that captures key information including age, gender, race, comorbidities, site where participant was recruited from, date of signed consent, serious adverse events, endpoints, and study completion (or early termination) date. Creation and implementation of the spreadsheet will improve efficiency by providing information for generating progress reports to the site's regulatory board or sponsor and extracting data to track participants for callbacks and future studies.

SUMMARY

Designing and implementing recruitment and retention strategies is critical to successful conduct and completion of clinical trials. Clinical investigators should be proactive in creating study-specific strategies well in advance of study launch. Including anticipated recruitment tools in study protocol submitted to the investigator's regulatory board will save time and energy. Meeting with study team members prior to and during the conduct of the study, on a regular basis, to evaluate recruitment and retention strategies and measure the performance of such strategies will ensure that the study is completed successfully.

How to Set up Your Database

Janet P. Smith, BA

INTRODUCTION

Although the concepts in this chapter can be applied to any database project—planning, defining, developing, executing, monitoring, reviewing, analyzing, and reporting—it is important to recognize that there are special considerations in applying these to a medical research project (1–3). These include regulatory and reporting requirements, review boards, randomization, study subject confidentiality, and audit trails. Since studies are similar, in that they follow a protocol with predefined time points, certain techniques can be applied in the design phase that will assist in the creation of a well-organized database which not only will house the study data but will be easy to query to provide data and reports for analysis, study subject tracking, quality control, monitoring, and for regulatory and other reporting agencies.

When building a study team, including both an experienced database professional and a biostatistician will provide the requisite expertise for appropriate statistical design, sample size estimates, budgetary estimates, forms design, database development, randomization methods, data management, and reporting. A professional database designer knows that certain concepts are essential for the organization of a database. Involving a designer early in the process will ensure that essential elements are included that will guarantee proper organization. This can prevent problems later on that might cause project delays necessitating an expensive re-do.

DATA DEFINITION AND FORMS DESIGN

Visual aids, such as charts, a list of specific information needed to define data items, and suggestions for forms, can assist team members in proceeding from the initial planning to successful implementation of a study.

Identify What Data Elements Are to be Collected and When They Will be Collected

A study proposal states the goals of the study, methods, and outcome measures. A protocol schedule gives a visual summary representation of the project. It describes an event time line and the data collected. Time points are specifically defined and have a designation such as "Screening Visit" and "Study Visit 1." Tasks to be completed and data to be collected are associated with each time point. This representation assists in identifying forms for the project. An example of a protocol schedule is shown in **Table 9-1**.

Hint: It is easier to look at a chart than to read paragraphs of descriptive text. Making a protocol schedule into a chart is a first step toward being organized.

Make a List of Forms

Case report forms link the data items to be collected and the study database. The design of these forms is critical to the success of the project. Things to consider when creating these forms include who will fill out a form, where it will be filled out, when the data will be available, and whether the form will be part of the study database. By allocating data according to these criteria, individual forms can be identified.

Forms can be useful in ways other than listing study data. They can assist in reporting, tracking, study logistics, and quality control. For example, the pharmacy may need a "Randomization Request" form that will provide the information necessary for randomization and dosage. A "Forms Check-List" helps organize a study and tracks the forms to ensure that all are completed. A "Study subject ID Assignment Log" can be used to give an anonymous identifier to a study subject. An "Exit from Study" form records when a study subject leaves the study, completion status, and the reason. **Table 9-2** lists typical forms that could be used in a study.

Describe Data Elements to be Collected

Understanding the data to be collected is necessary for the design of a good form. Each item should be carefully defined. Often, important procedural issues for the study are brought up and can be addressed *before* the start of the study. For each data item, the investigator should ask these questions:

1. What is the description of the item?
2. How is it measured? (Evaluate the need for written instructions, personnel training, reliability testing, special equipment, an expert consultant.)
3. What is the data type? (numeric, date, text, true/false)
4. What are the units? (e.g., lbs, cm)

TABLE 9-1 | Example of a Protocol Schedule

| | Initial Contact | Screening | | Visit | | | | | Number of Times Measured |
		S1 Day 1	S2	V1 1 Month	V2 3 Months	V3 6 Months	V4 9 Months	V5 12 Months	
Pre-enrollment	X								1
Study subject number assignment	X								1
Inclusion/exclusion criteria		X							1
Informed consent		X							1
Study subject contact information		X							1
Medical history		X							1
Physical exam		X		X	X	X	X	X	6
Concomitant medications		X		X	X	X	X	X	6
Laboratory data		X		X	X	X	X	X	6
Randomization		X							
Start drug			X						
Drug adherence				X	X	X			3
Stop drug						X			
Study subject exit from study									At any time
Adverse event									As needed
Serious adverse event									As needed
Protocol violation									As needed

This chart lists time points in an example protocol (day 1, 1 month, 3 months, etc.) with a coding designation (S1, S2, V1, V2, etc.) to sort time points in the database. The "X" indicates when an event occurs and which form is filled out.

TABLE **9-2** | **Typical Study Forms**

External to Study Database	For Study Database
Study subject ID assignment log	Pre-enrollment
Signed consent	Inclusion/exclusion criteria
Study subject contact information	Randomization request
Study subject diary	Medical history
	Physical exam/vital signs
	Laboratory results
	Concomitant medications
Used for logistics	Drug dose assignment/adherence
Pharmacy request	Exit from Study
Forms checklist	Adverse event
Data entry request	Serious adverse event
	Protocol violation

Study forms can be used not only for collecting study data for analysis, but also to help the study run smoothly. Some forms are not entered into the study database.

5. What is the format? (e.g., number of digits, decimal places)
6. What is the expected range and what are acceptable values? (Define codes and lookup tables, how to indicate missing, refused, not applicable. Define data validation rules.)
7. How will data be obtained? (keying, image, instrumentation)
8. How will data be used? (analysis, information, logistics, reporting)

Answering these questions may prompt other details that need to be included in the implementation plan. For example, if special equipment or a new procedure will be used, allow for personnel training. For a critical outcome variable, evaluate the need for assessing reliability.

With the information above, a data dictionary can be created. This is usually developed by the forms designer or database developer. These experts know when to use codes (and lookup tables) to make data more reliable, consistent, and easier to enter and analyze. (An example of coding is 1 = yes, 0 = no, 8 = refused, 9 = unknown.) A sample data dictionary is shown in **Table 9-3**.

Hint: After the data dictionary is created, you are well on the way toward a goal of well-defined data for analysis. BUT, first the data have to be captured.

Design the Forms

The following guidelines will help produce an easy-to-use form.
Every data collection form needs a header. See **Figure 9-1** for an example of a form header.

- Name of the study
- Grant or study number
- Principal investigator (PI) name(s)
- Form title

T A B L E **9-3** | **Example of Items in a Data Dictionary**

Database Data Item Name	Description	Type	Format	Validation
Gender	Study subject's gender 1 = male 2 = female	Numeric	x	Lookup table
Visit_type	Type of visit S = screening V = protocol visit	Text	x	Lookup table
Visit_date	Date of visit	Date	mm/dd/yyyy	Valid date
A1C	Hemoglobin A1C (%)	Numeric	x.x	
PFTExMax	Maximal expiratory pressure in one second (cm/H_2O)	Numeric	xxx	<150
WBC	White blood cell count	Numeric	xx.xx	

A data dictionary gives necessary information about each variable stored in the database. It is an invaluable tool for defining a database as well as querying for reports and analyses. In the table above, X represents how many digits or characters a data item requires.

- Page number if more than one page
- Identifiers to *uniquely* identify a filled-in form
- Date collected

The most important header items are the identifiers. The combination of identifiers must provide a *unique* set of information that tie a paper form to a specific record in the database. To make a correction in the database, or find a paper form that goes with a specific record, the identifiers link the two. The identifiers can also be utilized to put data in sequence for analysis.

Examples of unique identifiers:

Center #, Study Subject #, Visit Type, Visit #
Center #, Study Subject #, Date
Study Subject #, Treatment Day #

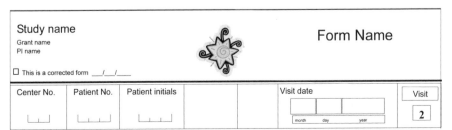

FIGURE **9-1**   Example of a form header. A form header provides continuity of design for all forms in a study. It should identify the study, investigator, grant number, form name, and give a set unique identifiers, shown in the bottom row, that link the form and the record in the database.

A site identifier (Center #) is needed for a multicenter study. The Study Subject # is an identifier assigned to the study subject and comes from the "Study Subject Number Assignment Log" form. In addition, using study subject initials gives a way to double check that the Study Subject # belongs to the correct study subject. Date of visit or event and, depending on the study, time-of-day are important to capture. If the protocol has fixed time points, then visit 1, visit 2, or visit 3 should be designated. Compare the two forms shown in **Figures 9-2 and 9-3**. Both forms capture the same information, but form 2 is better designed:

- Numbering items makes it clear what the questions are and provides a handy reference for discussions and documentation and facilitates data entry.
- Sections, dividing lines, and boxes make it easier to locate a specific item on the form. Notice the three shaded sections and the box around the answers for item 4. (If shading is used, make sure it is light enough to copy well.)
- Showing formats and units will make it clear what is expected. Notice age on Form 1 does not specify units, while on Form 2, age is specified as months. On Form 1, date of pre-enrollment contact does not show format; header items do not show number of characters. On Form 2, formats of header items are designated. Other examples showing formats and units are

Lab value _ _ _ . _ mg/dc
Weight _ _ _ . _ kg

- Use of check boxes and inclusion of corresponding database codes is shown on Form 2. On Form 1, gender could get any number of responses: "M", "Male", "F", "Female", "Fem." There would be no consistency of data in the database. Using the database codes shown on Form 2, the data entry operator can simply enter the code for the response checked. This ensures only valid data values enter the database.
- Providing instructions for check boxes ("check all that apply" or "check one") will help prevent misunderstanding by the person filling out the form.
- Most items with choices should allow for an "other" response with sufficient space to describe it.

Other Design Considerations

- Think about how missing data will be reflected in the database. If an item on the form is blank, is it because the item had missing data or was the item skipped? Is there a need to designate "not done" or "not applicable"? For the missing reason responses, use codes such as "99" or "–9," or anything that would not be confused with real data values.
- Avoid double negatives
  - Confusing: "Do **not** enroll study subject if above criteria are **not** met."
  - Better: "Enroll the study subject if all the above criteria are met."
- Link actions to individuals, so responsibilities are clear.
  - Unclear: "Permission for the next level of dosing can be obtained when lab results are provided."
  - Clear: "Send the lab results to the Study Monitor, who will inform you if the study subject can proceed to next level of dosing."
- Break down compound questions into single-idea questions.

Study Name
Grant number
PI name

Pre-Enrollment

Center No.	Patient No.	Patient initials			Date of pre-enrollment contact	

Age: _____   Patient's Zip Code (1st 3 digits): _____

Ethnic Category   __ Hispanic or Latino   __ Not Hispanic or Latino   __ Unknown

Racial Category   __ American Indian/ Alaskan Native   __ Asian
                     __ Black or African American __ Native Hawaiian or Other Pacific Islander
                     __ White __ More than one race
                     __ Unknown or not reported

English speaking?   __ Yes __ No

Native Language: _____

Translator present?   __ Yes __ No

Gender: _____

Mode of contact   __ Phone   __ Letter   __ In clinic   __ Other

Who initiated contact?   __ Patient   __ Referring physician   __ Clinic staff   __ Other

How did you first hear about the study?
          __ Referring physician   __ Family member
          __ Friend   __ Clinic staff
          __ Advertisement   __ Other

Was consent signed? (patient enrolled)   __ Yes __ No

If consent not signed, give primary reason. _____

Was drug dispensed?   __ Yes __ No

If not dispensed, give primary reason: _____

Coordinator signature: _____   Date: _____

FIGURE **9-2**   Form example 1. This form, although neat in appearance, leaves some items open to misinterpretation and may result in unusable data.

- Avoid abbreviations and medical terms if the person completing the form may not understand what is meant.
  - A mystery: "H/O"; better: "history of."
  - A mystery: "SOB"; better: "shortness of breath."
- More pages in the form are better than crowded forms.

Study Name
Grant number
PI name

Pre-Enrollment

Center No.	Patient No.	Patient initials			Date of pre-enrollment contact
⊔_⊔	⊔_⊔_⊔	⊔_⊔_⊔			month day year

PATIENT INFORMATION

1. Patient Age (months): ⊔_⊔   2. Patient's Zip Code (1st 3 digits): ⊔_⊔_⊔

3. Ethnic Category (check one) ☐₁ Hispanic or Latino   ☐₂ Not Hispanic or Latino   ☐₃ Unknown

4. Racial Category (check one)
   - ☐₁ American Indian/ Alaskan Native   ☐₄ Asian
   - ☐₂ Black or African American   ☐₅ Native Hawaiian or Other Pacific Islander
   - ☐₃ White   ☐₆ More than one race
                                           ☐₇ Unknown or not reported

5. English speaking?   ☐₁ Yes ☐₀ No

6. Native Language: _____

7. Translator present?   ☐₁ Yes ☐₀ No

8. Gender: ☐₁ Male ☐₂ Female

CONTACT

9. Mode of contact (check one)   ☐₁ Phone   ☐₂ Letter   ☐₃ In clinic   ☐₄ Other _____

10. Who initiated contact?   ☐₁ Patient ☐₂ Referring physician ☐₃ Clinic staff ☐₄ Other _____

11. How did you first hear about the study? (check one)
    - ☐₁ Referring physician   ☐₄ Family member
    - ☐₂ Friend   ☐₅ Clinic staff
    - ☐₃ Advertisement   ☐₆ Other _____

ENROLLMENT

12. Was consent signed? (patient enrolled)   ☐₁ Yes ☐₀ No

13. If consent not signed, give primary reason. _____

14. Was drug dispensed?   ☐₁ Yes ☐₀ No

15. If not dispensed, give primary reason. _____

Coordinator signature: _____   Date: _____

Pre-Enroll
rev 08/19/2008

FIGURE **9-3**   Form example 2. This form is more specific about what is expected than form example 1. It numbers items and organizes data into sections, uses checkboxes with entry codes, and defines formats and units.

- Use upper and lower case text for readability.
- Use standardized coding, if possible (e.g., ICD-9 codes).
- If collecting time of day, always include the date.
- Spacing:
  - ○ Less space shows items that are related.
  - ○ More space separates unrelated items.
- Margins: Allow for hole punching, binding.
- Include places for signatures and comments.
- Include a version number and date of form revision at the bottom of the form.

Implementation Suggestions

- Pilot test forms. Have other experts review and critique the form design. If possible, use them to collect "real" data and compare answers with expectations. Revise forms accordingly.
- Keep a history of changes to the forms with date of change and version number.

Hint: Careful analysis and planning along with the use of tools such as a protocol schedule and data dictionary will lead to well-defined data. Using techniques for good forms design will result in clear easy-to-use forms and more reliable data in the database.

DATA COLLECTION AND MANAGEMENT PLAN

Activities to be addressed in a plan are managing case report forms, mechanism of data entry, managing lab specimens, study subject tracking, identifying and managing discrepancies, creating reports, transferring data, ensuring quality control and security.

The plan should be formulated early in the project. Identify work to be performed: who is responsible for each task, what quality control checks to incorporate, what is the flow of study subjects and data, what procedures or guidelines apply, what documentation to collect, and what output to generate.

Common sources of errors can be attributed to poor form design, lack of written definitions and procedures leading to inconsistent interpretation, improperly made observations, inaccurate measuring devices, protocol violations, protocol deviations, improperly entered data, and inadequate security. Address these when making the plan. The first objective is to prevent errors; the next is to be able to identify and address them in a timely manner. No researcher wants to find out at the end of the study that data are missing or incorrect. Having a robust database will make problem solving easier by providing reports of study subject accrual, adverse events, withdrawals, timeliness of CRF submissions, overdue visits, missing data, and cross-check errors.

Hint: Think ahead about how you will ensure reliable data for analysis.

DATABASE SELECTION AND DESIGN

Depending on its complexity, a study may only need a simple means to collect data; multisite or longitudinal studies will need a more sophisticated approach.

Example of a Table in a Database

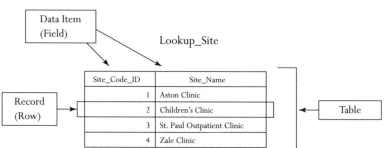

FIGURE **9-4** Example of a table. This shows a lookup table that contains two data items: the code used for the site and the name of the site. The code is stored in the data records. The names are displayed in drop-down choices during data entry and on reports.

What Is a Database, Anyway?

A database is a collection of related data stored in a structured format. One can think of a database as the container of study data. Many researchers believe that Excel is a database. In fact, Excel is a popular vehicle for accruing data and can be used for simple studies with only a few data items (4). However, a true database has the adjective "relational" associated with it. Examples of relational database software products are Microsoft Access, Microsoft SQL, and Oracle. Imbedded in the database are "tables" with "records" and "indices" **(Figure 9-4)**. A table is a container of like-defined records (study subject demographics, study subject visits). An index is a separate structure, managed by the software, which allows quick access to a record based on an identifier or identifiers without searching all the records in the table. The advantage of a relational database is that common identifiers can be used to "match" and access data in other tables. For example, a database query can produce a list of study subjects and their visits by using PID (study subject identifier) in the study subject table and visit table to relate the data.

Hint: Excel cannot relate records; but information entered in Excel spreadsheets can be imported into a relational database such as Access.

Database Organization

A hierarchal design within a relational database is the best way to organize a typical research study database **(Figure 9-5)**. The main table ("Study subjects") has one record for each subject. It contains information such as site (if multisite study), ethnicity, gender, and the anonymous study subject identifier that was assigned in the "Study Subject Number Assignment Log." The unique record identifier (primary key) denoted as PID is a software-generated number not dependent on any data variable, an approach that simplifies internal organization and querying of the database.

Next in the hierarchy is a table, "Study Subject Visits." It has a primary key denoted as VID (a software generated number), but it also contains the PID to relate the visit to the study subject. Key items in this table are the "Visit Number" which identifies where the visit

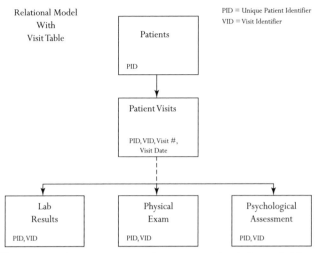

Relational Model
With
Visit Table

PID = Unique Patient Identifier
VID = Visit Identifier

FIGURE 9-5   Study database organization. This is an example of a hierarchal design in a relational database. It organizes data to identify each study subject and each visit during the study, and all forms associated with a particular visit. The identifiers PID and VID are used to relate the data. The inclusion of the visit table ensures queries will produce correct results.

fits in the protocol (e.g., S1 meaning Screening Visit 1) and the visit date. It can also hold other data that are needed on a visit level. Think of this table as a "place holder" for all forms collected on a visit.

When forms are entered for a protocol visit (e.g., lab results, physical exam, results of psychological assessments), each will be stored in its respective table, using PID to relate to the "Study Subjects" table and VID to relate to the "Study Subject Visits" table. Each table can also hold a date if it is different from that in the "Study Subject Visits" table. To maintain database integrity, a study subject record and visit record must exist before any form is entered for a visit for that study subject. These tables reside in the lowest level of the hierarchy.

Unfortunately, many novices use an inadequate design and omit the "Study Subject Visits" table, thinking it is unnecessary, and instead, store visit number and visit date in each form's record. The reason this design is problematic has to do with how queries work in a database. As shown in the example protocol schedule, certain measures are not collected at every visit, and some measures may have been collected on a different date from another measure's date, yet belong to the same visit. The novice designer will think that one can simply relate, for example, labs to physical exam and psychological assessment results, based on PID and visit number or on PID and dates. This will not produce the desired results and will omit records **(Figure 9-6)**. How would you query such a database to get a list of all study subjects and all their visit dates? How would you know that the data entry person entered an incorrect visit number in one of the records? By using the additional "Study Subject Visits" table in the hierarchy, one can reliably query the database **(Figure 9-7)**.

Relational database software is utilized to define data formats and data validations. The software provides the facility to generate ad hoc queries and display data from a query in a

List Hachinski Score and MMS Score for all patient visits.

Table: Hachinski

Patient ID	HachDate	HachScore
1001	9/15/2004	10
1001	1/15/2005	8
1001	4/15/2005	9
2002	9/25/2004	11
2002	11/1/2004	10
2002	3/12/2005	9

Table: Mini Mental Status Exam

Patient ID	MMSDate	MMSScore	
1001	9/15/2004	18	
1001	10/2/2004	27	← missed
1001	1/15/2005	20	
1001	4/15/2005	21	
2002	9/25/2004	28	
2002	3/12/2005	21	

Relating records on Patient ID and Date will not return all records.
(Include all records in Hachinski and those that match in Mini Mental)

Patient ID	HachDate	HachScore	MMSDate	MMSScore	
1001	9/15/2004	10	9/15/2004	18	
1001	1/15/2005	8	1/15/2005	20	6 records instead of 7
1001	4/15/2005	9	4/15/2005	21	
2002	9/25/2004	11	9/25/2004	28	
2002	11/1/2004	10			
2002	3/12/2005	9	3/12/2005	21	

FIGURE **9-6**   Unsuccessful query. This database does not have a visit table. Thus there is no way to find all the records when there is missing data in any of the tables.

List Hachinski Score and MMS Score for all patient visits.

Table: Hachinski

Patient ID	Visit Nbr	HachScore
1001	1	10
1001	3	8
1001	4	9
2002	1	11
2002	2	10
2002	3	9

Table: Visits

Patient ID	Visit Nbr	Visit Date
1001	1	9/15/2004
1001	2	10/2/2004
1001	3	1/15/2005
1001	4	4/15/2005
2002	1	9/25/2004
2002	2	11/1/2004
2002	3	3/12/2005

Table: Mini Mental Status Exam

Patient ID	Visit Nbr	MMSScore
1001	1	18
1001	2	27
1001	3	20
1001	4	21
2002	1	28
2002	3	21

Relating records using Patient ID and Visit Nbr from the Visit Table will find all records.
(Include all records in Visit Table and those that match in other tables.)

Patient ID	Visit Nbr	Visit Date	HachScore	MMSScore	
1001	1	9/15/2004	10	18	
1001	2	10/2/2004		27	7 records
1001	3	1/15/2005	8	20	
1001	4	4/15/2005	9	21	
2002	1	9/25/2004	11	28	
2002	2	11/1/2004	10		
2002	3	3/12/2005	9	21	

FIGURE **9-7**   Successful query. This database includes a visit table and successfully finds all the records. This is because the visit table has no missing data.

report or export it for use in a statistical program. Database products such as Microsoft Access have a programming language to incorporate the checking that is desired. Other features include security and multiuser capability.

Hint: You need a database developer to implement these features.

QUALITY CONTROL IN DATA CAPTURE

Use of a computer can add quality control features to data capture. **Figure 9-8** shows a generic flow of data from capture to analysis. Data may come into the computer in several ways—manual data entry to a local server or over the Web, scanning, and transfer from another database or device. A well-designed system will provide appropriate validations and error checks at each step. For example, if manual data entry is used, there is an important increase in reliability of data if case report forms are entered twice by two different people (double data entry). Properly designed forms can limit the responses to each question (1 = yes, 0 = no) or impose numerical range checks as the data are entered. More comprehensive checks can be done after the data are in the database. These should involve comparisons across forms or visits, looking for missing data and inconsistencies, and producing error reports for review. Scanned data should be subjected to checks by the scanner operator or a computer checking program before it is merged into a database.

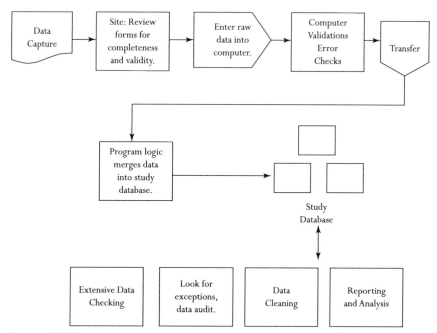

FIGURE **9-8**   Generic flow of data. Data checking should occur at various points during the time from data capture to finalization for analysis. It should be done both by people and by the computer.

DATABASES AND SECURITY

There are three aspects of security that form the "Security Triad": Confidentiality—protection of data from unauthorized viewing; Integrity—ensuring data accuracy; and Availability—ensuring accessibility by authorized users. The security triad is used as an industry standard (5) and can be applied to clinical trials.

Confidentiality deals with making sure that only authorized and authenticated individuals or processes access study data. Examples are keeping forms in locked cabinets, using encryption on laptops and other mobile devices, password protecting computers and databases, never leaving a workstation without locking it, never leaving passwords in obvious places, and using complex passwords. A study database should only contain "de-identified" study subject data, as stated in the "Health Insurance Portability and Accountability Act of 1996 (HIPAA) Privacy Rule" guidelines regarding study subject protected information (6).

Integrity deals with making sure that data elements are not inappropriately altered, either intentionally or accidentally. Levels of security can be incorporated into a database, such as read/only access, update ability, full access. Each user would be given access rights according to the function they perform. For example, a developer would have full access, a data entry person would have limited update ability, and an investigator might have read/only access for querying.

Availability deals with making sure that data are available when needed. The "users" of the database include the database manager/coordinator, data entry personnel, and the statistician for the project as well as other project personnel (investigator, coordinator, etc.). In addition, availability also includes backup, restoration, recovery, and redundancy of the database.

Computers and networks need protection from intrusions over the Web. It is imperative that an organization implement technical safeguards such as firewalls and virus protection. It is best to house study data on a protected server that has regular backups. However, one must consider the possibility that data could also reside on laptops or other external devices. Encryption is highly recommended for these devices in case of theft or loss. Other considerations include administrative safeguards defined in policies and procedures, electronic access logs, sign-in sheets, and physical safeguards such as secure servers and workstations and limited access to secure areas.

THE IMPORTANCE OF AN AUDIT TRAIL

The FDA definition of an audit trail in their Guidance for Industry—Computerized Systems Used in Clinical Trials is, "*Audit Trail* means, for the purposes of this guidance, a secure, computer generated, time-stamped electronic record that allows reconstruction of the course of events relating to the creation, modification, and deletion of an electronic record" (7).

Although, this statement describes electronic audit trails, the concept should be expanded to include paper as well. Most important is modification of study data. Perhaps a change is needed after a cross-check report turns up an inconsistency. Not only should the change be notated on the paper case report form with date and initials of the person making the change, but a formal request should be submitted to authorize the data manager to modify the database. Separate documents should be maintained to describe the addition/deletion of data items, changes in definition, and changes to procedures, forms, or protocol. Documentation should describe who made the change, and when and why it was made. This is the responsibility of the database designer or project coordinator.

Maintaining an audit trail is good practice and not only satisfies regulations, but also provides an invaluable tool for data queries and questions that arise during analysis.

DATA CLEANING AND LOCK

Data cleaning is a process of examination, research, and correction or certification of questionable data. As discussed earlier, coded data with choices stated on a case report form will be validated during data entry and only valid codes will enter the database. Other checks must be handled after data are in the database. The specifications for the checking program must be defined by the investigator in collaboration with the database analyst and biostatistician. Problems that should be reported are missing values for critical variables, out-of-range measurements (e.g., laboratory results, height, weight, age), and inconsistency in data across forms or across visits (e.g., study subject category changes from one visit to another). The checking program will produce a report and after review will result in either a correction to the database (and case report form) or a statement that the error has been reviewed and data are acceptable as is and should not appear on future reports. It is best to run the checking protocol at frequent intervals during the course of the study. This allows questions to be researched and corrections to be made close to the time the data were collected. Unfortunately many studies do not undergo this scrutiny and problems do not surface until the statistical analysis phase.

A final cleaning and checking should be done at the end of the study. This assumes all study subjects have completed the protocol or are otherwise accounted for, and all data forms have been received and entered. During this period, a "soft lock" or "freeze" should be imposed on the database. This is a controlled time period in which thorough checking is done to make sure all forms are entered, all discrepancies are accounted for, and all corrections are in the database. This is also a good time to check for unexpected results, such as outliers. The biostatistician may uncover other problems during preliminary analysis. Only supervisory personnel and their designees have access to the database. If the database needs updating, it will be temporarily unlocked to make the changes.

After cleaning, the data are ready for final analysis and a copy of the database is made for the statistician. When analyses are complete and no other problems are found, "final lock" or "permanent freeze" will be imposed in which access authorization will be removed from the database and no further changes will be allowed.

The statistician should retain a copy of the database that was used in the analysis along with documentation of queries and routines that were used to produce the results. This allows reproducibility after the fact. It is not uncommon for questions to come up when articles are submitted, sometimes many months after the completion of the study.

SUMMARY

A number of areas to address to ensure a successful study database have been discussed. Even with all the planning and careful execution, human error can still be a factor. Therefore it is essential that responsible detail-oriented people with the appropriate expertise are part of the research team. Do not take anything for granted. Have checks in place throughout the life cycle of the study.

REFERENCES

1. McFadden E. *Management of Data in Clinical Trials.* Hoboken, NJ: John Wiley & Sons, Inc; 2007.
2. Prokscha S. *Practical Guide to Clinical Data Management.* 2nd ed. Boca Raton, FL: CRC Press; 2007.
3. Rondel R, Varley S, Webb C. *Clinical Data Management.* 2nd ed. West Sussex, England: John Wiley & Sons Ltd; 2002.
4. Elliott A, Hynan L, Reisch J, et al. Preparing data for analysis using Microsoft Excel. *J Invest Med.* 2006;54(6):334–341.
5. The CIA Triad. http://blogs.techrepublic.com.com/security/?p=488.
6. The Health Insurance Portability and Accountability Act of 1996 (HIPAA) Privacy Rule. http://www.hhs.gov/ocr/privacy/.
7. U.S. Food and Drug Administration Guidance for Industry—Computerized Systems Used in Clinical Trials. http://www.fda.gov/RegulatoryInformation/Guidances/ucm126402.htm.

CHAPTER 10

Budgeting Process and Management

Deanna S. Adams, RN

OUTLINE

INTRODUCTION

The development, management, and monitoring of a protocol budget are key activities in the conduct of clinical research. Without sufficient funding, an investigator will be unable to complete the necessary activities to answer the research questions and accomplish the objectives of the protocol. In contrast, if the budget is too large, it may be impossible to find a funding source that will support the proposed research. For the purpose of this chapter, elements of the budget are organized chronologically from the time that the investigator begins to develop a research proposal, or receives a protocol from a sponsor. The National Institutes of Health (NIH) form PHS 398 used for filing grant submissions uses the terms Direct Costs for the line items that comprise a proposed protocol budget. The form can be found on the NIH website at this link: http://grants.nih.gov/grants/funding/phs398/phs398.html. Direct Costs are the budgeted amounts that will be required for the conduct of the proposed research **(Table 10-1)**. The NIH provides descriptions and instructions for the costs to be included in each of these categories (Appendix H).

However, the total of the direct costs of conducting the research may not be reflected by simply covering each of these areas. The investigator will need to consider the costs of each element of the research, each research-related activity, and the time required, then organize the information appropriately into the format required by the funding source.

THE FUNDING SOURCE

It is important for the investigator to know what is allowed by the funding source that is providing the money to conduct the research. While some grants may be unrestricted, these are becoming increasingly rare in the current economic climate.

NIH Cooperative Group Protocols

NIH Cooperative Group protocols will typically request a budget proposal from the investigator based on the costs to conduct the research at the investigator's institution. Since many of these protocols meet Medicare and Medicaid coverage guidelines for the payment

TABLE **10-1** | Direct Costs

1. Personnel
2. Consultant costs
3. Equipment
4. Supplies
5. Travel
6. Patient care costs, if any
7. Alterations and renovations
8. Other expenses

of research-related costs, the investigator (his/her institution) will be able to bill most of the subject costs to the subjects' third-party payers **(Table 10-2)**. However, the investigator will need to assure that those costs that are not directly billable are covered adequately by the proposed budget.

T A B L E **10-2** | **Guidance for the Public, Industry, and CMS Staff, National Coverage Determinations with Data Collection as a Condition of Coverage: Coverage with Evidence Development, Document Issued on July 12, 2006**

Research Studies

If Centers for Medicare and Medicaid Services (CMS) determines that the evidence for coverage of certain items or services is inadequate to establish Medicare coverage under 1862(a)(1)(A), Medicare may still reimburse for that item or service for Medicare beneficiaries enrolled in a research study that provides data and information to be used to evaluate that item or service as well as reimburse for the routine costs incurred by Medicare beneficiaries in the study.

To qualify for reimbursement, such a study must be designed to produce evidence that could be used in a future national coverage decision that would focus on whether the item or service should be covered by Medicare under 1862(a)(1)(A). Payment for the items and services provided in the study will be restricted to the Medicare-qualified patients involved as human subjects in the study.

CMS will not routinely be involved in the design, review, or execution of research studies. CMS will only provide payment for clinical research that meets the standards of a qualified trial as will be outlined in the revision of the Clinical Trial Policy. We anticipate this National Coverage Determination (NCD) will include the following principles:

1. The primary purpose of the trial is to test whether the intervention potentially improves the participants' health outcomes.
2. The trial is well supported by available scientific and medical information or is intended to clarify or establish the health outcomes of interventions already in common clinical use.
3. The trial does not duplicate existing studies unjustifiably.
4. The trial design is appropriate to answer the research question being asked in the trial.
5. The trial is sponsored by a credible organization or individual capable of executing the proposed trial successfully.
6. The trial is in compliance with Federal regulations relating to the protection of human subjects.
7. All aspects of the trial are conducted according to the appropriate standards of scientific integrity.
8. The trial is listed in the National Library of Medicine clinical trials database.
9. The sample of study subjects in the trial should include individuals representative of the Medicare population with the condition described in the NCD.

Industry-Sponsored Protocols

Industry-sponsored protocols often have a predetermined budget. The sponsor is supplying the study drug or device, any necessary equipment, a central laboratory for testing, etc. The sponsor provides the investigator with a simple list of the amounts that will be paid for certain research-related activities, as listed above. More commonly, the sponsor will simply propose a payment per subject (or per visit). In these situations, the investigator must calculate a budget for the protocol based on costs for the supporting services necessary to conduct the protocol and assure that the sponsor's proposed amounts will provide adequate payment.

An investigator may propose an idea to an industry sponsor utilizing the sponsor's drug or device for a new indication, or comparing different drugs or devices approved for the same diagnosis. For this type of research, the investigator must prepare a budget and seek funding from the company. In most cases, the company does not want to be considered a sponsor for the protocol.

Grant-Funded Research

Research that will be funded by a grant presents a continuum of possibilities for the investigator. NIH grants (RO-1, K grants, T grants and similar, Requests for Proposals [RFP]) will be submitted using the required (electronic) format using the budget sections listed above. Detailed justification must be provided for each of the proposed expenses.

Numerous institutes, foundations, government agencies, and community organizations have funds available for the conduct of clinical research. These grants will be funded based on the investigator's budget proposal, after any necessary justification and negotiation. However, some of these funding sources have restrictions on what may be paid; for example, travel may be specifically excluded, or limited.

Others may provide only a specified amount for a particular area of research (e.g., $5000 for a study of family violence) and assume the investigator has access to the necessary infrastructure to conduct the research with the funds provided.

PRELIMINARY COSTS

The preliminary costs as described here are the costs associated with the development and conduct of a research protocol apart from the costs directly related to the research subject.

Development Costs

These are the costs associated with the development of the protocol and determining what data will need to be collected and how often subjects will need to be seen.

Preliminary Research

For some projects, a simple data collection study can be a cost-effective way to obtain information about the feasibility of the proposed research, the available subject population, local standard care treatments, and other data that will inform the design of the protocol. See Chapter 12 on collecting data for additional information on this subject.

Biostatistician

Unless the investigator is qualified in this discipline, most protocols will require the services of a biostatistician. The design of the protocol, data elements, and methods of data analysis are just a sample of the services that may be provided. While an academic medical center may provide consultation with a biostatistician free of charge, investigators in hospital or private practice settings may need to include the fees for this service in the protocol budget.

Bioinformatics/Software

As facilities adopt various electronic medical record (EMR) systems to comply with federal mandates, the ability of the investigator to interact with and utilize these systems is critical to accomplishing clinical research. Many of these systems have research modules that are designed to meet the needs of the investigator. However, not all systems have this capability, and not all institutions have elected to use the research modules, even when they are available.

Working with a bioinformatics specialist would be the ideal for most investigators, but this service is often unavailable, except in larger, urban academic medical centers. These experts can assist the investigator in the development of data collection tools, spreadsheets, and electronic case report forms.

In the absence of EMR support or bioinformatics, the investigator will need to obtain commercial software that meets the needs of his/her study. This will entail both the cost of the software and any licensing fees. There will be further expenses if commercial software must be modified to meet the needs of the research.

Expert Consultation

The investigator may need the guidance of a more experienced clinician (a supervising physician or mentor) with whom to discuss the proposed research. While this type of guidance is expected in the academic environment, an investigator working in a hospital or private practice may need to pay for this type of knowledge and support.

Space

All research requires the use of some type of space, whether an inpatient bed, outpatient area, clinic, or office. Most institutions can provide a cost per square foot that can be used to calculate the investigator's financial responsibility for the use of a particular space during the time required for the research. In most cases, the cost per square foot includes utilities, maintenance, and housekeeping. It may also include basic equipment, for instance a treatment room with an exam table, or an office with a desk and chair. It does not usually include staff time, specialized equipment, telephone/fax, or accommodate high electrical usage; these will cost additional monies. See Chapter 7 on screening and evaluation for additional information on how much space is needed.

Inpatient

Inpatient research is usually the most expensive. If a study drug, device, or procedure requires inpatient hospitalization, the investigator will need to work with hospital administration to obtain a negotiated daily rate (per diem). Establish a clear understanding of what is included in that per diem. Room, bed, meals, and nursing care are standard. Ancillaries such as medications, supplies, laboratory tests, imaging procedures, telemetry, or therapy services will generate additional cost. Special diets (other than those routinely prepared by the hospital dietary department) may be charged. Specialty units usually have higher per diem rates than general medical–surgical floors.

Note: For NIH-funded research, federal regulations prohibit a facility from charging more for research services than Medicare will pay. The facility may work with the investigator to calculate a Diagnosis-Related Group (DRG) reimbursement rate based on the diagnoses and procedures of the subjects enrolled in the research. DRG reimbursement is all-inclusive; the investigator will not be charged for ancillaries.

Outpatient

As mentioned above, charges for use of outpatient space in a hospital is often calculated on a cost per square foot. Some facilities may have an hourly charge for the space to allow the investigator to pay for the space only for the time that it is actually used. If the investigator will need staff services as well (nurse, phlebotomist), these services will generate additional charges.

Clinic/Office

The physician in private practice, either individually or in a group, will need to assure that the cost of the conduct of the research is covered by the protocol budget. For example, if office hours will be extended, if there will be a need to purchase new or additional equipment, or if office personnel will need to work additional hours, these expenses should be included.

Alterations and Renovations

If the available space is not configured or equipped to meet the needs of the research, the investigator will need to work with a contractor to identify any alterations or renovations that will be needed and the associated costs. For example, a large clinic space might need to be subdivided into offices and a treatment room. In general, a sponsor would not cover this type of expense, and the investigator will need to work with his administration, colleagues, or partners to determine whether the importance of the research justifies the proposed expense.

Staffing

In this section, the staffing costs are the costs associated with research-related activities other than direct time spent with subjects.

Investigator's Time

For the investigator, substantial time is spent in preparatory and administrative tasks. The investigator must develop the protocol (or read and discuss a sponsored protocol received from another source); prepare a grant submission and respond to all stipulations (where applicable); meet with colleagues and consultants to discuss the research proposal; attend an investigator's meeting; spend time with the sponsor or sponsor's representative for site initiation activities; educate staff on the protocol; read and sign documents (source, CRFs); evaluate laboratory reports, diagnostic tests, and adverse events; monitoring visits, and responsibility for all necessary reporting and treatment required for serious adverse events.

It may be difficult for the investigator to make an accurate determination of the time required for all of these activities (both for themselves and any coinvestigators) in addition to the time allotted for subject visits. If acceptable to the sponsor, the investigator might use a percentage of personal time/salary to budget this expense.

Research Staff (Nurse, Research Coordinator, Research Assistant, Data Analyst)

Research staff members also have many responsibilities associated with the conduct of a research protocol in addition to direct time with subjects. These may include preparation of regulatory documents; preparation and submission of IRB documents and responses to any stipulations, attending the investigators' meeting; spending time with the sponsor or sponsor's representative for site initiation activities; preparation of source documents; completion of CRFs; phone calls with subjects and monitors; monitoring visits and activities necessary to close the study. As previously noted for the investigator(s), it may be easier to calculate a percentage of time required for these activities.

If the protocol requires the addition of a new staff member, the investigator will need to work with Human Resources at the institution to determine the appropriate level of education, the required skill sets and the salary level for this position, then use the institution's Full Time Equivalent (FTE), usually 1.3 to 1.5 times the annual salary to allow for salary and benefits, to calculate the cost that will be included in the protocol budget.

Consultant Costs

For some studies, the investigator needs a particular type of knowledge or expertise that is not available in his/her research team or department. This might be for the administration of questionnaires, evaluations or ratings, or the interpretation of diagnostic tests (imaging or cardiology), or other study-specific activities. For example, in a protocol enrolling neonates, the investigator (a pediatrician/neonatologist) may need consultation services from a gynecologist regarding information obtained about the mother's pregnancy. In these situations, the investigator should negotiate a payment rate and payment schedule with the consultant and include this in the budget.

Capital Equipment

After personnel expenses, these can be the most expensive items in the protocol budget. If areas must be furnished, or if special equipment is necessary for the conduct of the research, the investigator will need to work with the institution's administration and approved vendors to obtain prices for the budget. Large hospitals and academic medical centers often have a stockpile of furniture, computers, and other types of equipment available. If used equipment is available, this would help to reduce cost.

For items that are rented, on multiyear protocols, the investigator will need to include the rental amounts for each year. In some cases, the monthly or annual rental rates may decrease as the value of the equipment depreciates.

Supplies

While the cost of individual supplies is small, the cost of these items can multiply quickly over the course of a protocol. Allowing adequate cost in the budget for these items can help to prevent budget overages.

Clinical Supplies

To estimate the cost of the clinical supplies needed, the investigator will need to review the research-related activities in the protocol and list the supplies needed to perform these tasks. These may be supplies to obtain blood and urine samples for laboratory tests, adhesive pads for electrocardiograms (EKG), supplies for IV administration, etc. Central Supply in the institution is the source for a complete price list of clinical supplies.

In some instances, the cost of a test or procedure may include all equipment, supplies, and staff time necessary to perform the test. For example, the charge for laboratory (blood) tests in a hospital usually comprises the services of the phlebotomist, the supplies necessary to draw the blood, and the processing of the test(s), and a hospital's EKG charge includes the EKG technician, the machine, and the electrodes and pads. The investigator will need to know what is included in the prices for the services that are needed.

Office Supplies

For office supplies (paper, pens, boxes of paper clips, binders, labels, etc.), most institutions can provide historical information regarding the annual purchase amounts for a department or division, which the investigator can use to estimate the cost over the life of his/her study.

Postage

While very little mailing, in the traditional sense, is necessary in this age of electronic communication, some things must still be shipped. Sponsors need original documents to meet regulatory requirements at the beginning of a protocol, for example the Food and Drug Administration (FDA) Form 1572. And some sponsors will require mailing of completed CRFs.

Laboratory specimens to be processed by a central laboratory must be sent to that laboratory, and the shipment of biohazardous materials is quite expensive. Special boxes, special packing materials, and dry ice may be needed. And such specimens must be shipped overnight to assure timely arrival and analysis.

For sponsored research, the sponsor pays for these items and supplies the necessary packaging, labels, etc. For investigator-initiated protocols, the investigator may need to compare rates and service from several vendors to obtain the optimum price. For example, some vendors may pick up shipments, while others require them to be dropped off at a location. How much will it cost to pay a member of the research team to deliver the shipment to the vendor's location?

Information Technology (Telephone, Computers, Printers, Copiers, and Fax Machines)

In most cases, this equipment must be purchased or rented, but the services necessary to operate the equipment will also need to be included in the protocol budget. There may also be charges for installation, maintenance, and repair of these machines. Below are some specific methods for estimating the costs of these items:

Telephone: allow for a basic monthly bill plus any additional charges required by the study, for example, long distance charges.

Computers: consider charges for the internet provider.

Printers, copiers and fax machines: allow appropriate amounts for the paper and ink or toner that will be necessary.

Large hospitals and academic medical centers have an Information Technology Department to work with the investigator on cost estimates for these services. Historical information may be available to provide a basis for budgeting.

Institutional Review Board

Most Institutional Review Boards (IRBs) charge a fee for their services, whether in a large hospital or academic medical center or central (commercial) board. These fees can range from several hundred to several thousand dollars, depending on the complexity of the protocol and the funding source for the research. On multicenter studies, each site will require separate IRB approval, and the IRB fee will be charged for each site.

Some IRBs have a sliding scale of fees depending on the funding source for the research. For example, for an initial review and approval, industry-sponsored research could be $1500, NIH-funded research at $500, and the fees waived for investigator-initiated research funded by NIH, a foundation grant or departmental funds.

In budgeting for IRB fees, the investigator needs to obtain the fee schedule for each service that the IRB will provide: initial approval, modifications, reporting of serious and unexpected adverse events (AE), and continuing reviews. These amounts need to be included in the budget. The investigator will need to estimate the numbers for modifications and AE reporting. Some IRBs also charge for reportable protocol violations; the investigator will need to be aware of this in the ongoing conduct of the research. Most commercial sponsors will allow the investigator to arrange direct billing to the sponsor (pass-through) for IRB fees.

Hospitals may also have compliance committees and approval processes in addition to IRB approval. There may be fees associated with the approval process, use of the hospital's resources or departmental fees. In particular, the pharmacy will usually charge setup fees, fees for drug storage and accountability activities, and fees for the time spent on study-related activities such as site initiation or monitoring visits.

Facilities and Administration (F&A) Fees

Large institutions charge the investigator an F&A Fee for the use of institutional resources in the conduct of a research protocol. Often considered facility overhead, the F&A Fee covers the facility's cost of doing business, including the personnel, physical plant, and services and supplies that are available to investigators. While this infrastructure enables investigators to perform clinical research without the significant costs associated with the creation of a research facility, these fees can be high and can significantly decrease the funds available for the actual research activities.

F&A fees are a percentage of the protocol budget. In a large academic medical center, F&A fees can range from as low of 10% for investigator-initiated research to as much as 60% for industry-sponsored or NIH cooperative group protocols. Typically, an institution will begin collecting the F&A percentage when the first payment is received and from each payment thereafter.

At some institutions (usually academic medical centers), there are F&A fees for research conducted on campus (as described above), and additional fees for research conducted at affiliated off-campus facilities. These additional fees may range from 5% to 26%. These rates and percentages are based on agreements with the Department of Health and Human Services (DHHS).

The investigator needs to be aware of everything that is covered by the facility's F&A fee, and especially aware of those things that are not included. At some institutions, nearly all of the costs previously mentioned in this section are included in the F&A. Some academic medical centers may also include clinical areas and the services of research personnel, if the institution has a grant that provides funding for those services. In other places, the F&A will only cover basic facility (office space, clinic) and administrative cost, and the investigator is expected to budget and obtain funding for everything else that is required for the conduct of the research.

Translation Services

If a protocol has potential benefit to subjects, most IRBs will require the investigator to enroll non-English-speaking subjects. IRBs have different policies for this. Some may approve a short-form Consent in the subject's language and the use of a translator during the consent process. Other boards may require a fully translated Consent or make the decision on a case-by-case basis depending on the complexity of the protocol. In any case, to satisfy the Justice principle as described in the Belmont Report, the investigator needs to make provision for the enrollment of non-English-speaking subjects, particularly if the community includes a large proportion of persons who do not speak or read English.

Translation services may be available through the investigator's hospital or institution. For the translation of documents (the Consent and any other forms required for research subjects), there may be a fee, often based on the number of words or per page. The services of a translator to participate in the consent process may also have an associated charge. The investigator will need to budget for these costs.

Travel

Preparing to initiate a protocol may involve travel for the investigator and also members of the research team. If the investigator is the principal investigator for a multicenter study, travel to other sites will certainly be necessary for site initiation, training, and monitoring activities. Most funding sources use the current government rates for mileage. If the protocol is sponsored or funded by NIH, most travel vendors (airfare lines, hotels, car rental companies) will give a government rate. The investigator will also need to be aware of his/her institution's per diem allowances for hotel, meals, etc. and stay within those limits.

Insurance

Consider the risk profile of the research and the likelihood that a subject will experience an adverse event that is directly or possibly related to participation in the protocol. Serious adverse events can quickly become expensive. For events that are clearly research related, the subject's insurance or third-party payer will not usually provide payment. The investigator may want to consider insurance to cover expenses related to treatment of research-related adverse events. For investigators in large hospitals or academic medical centers, a consultation with the institution's legal staff may be appropriate. Some organizations prefer not to have insurance in place for research protocols.

COSTS OF CONDUCTING A RESEARCH PROTOCOL

The first step to determining the costs of conducting a human research protocol is the development of a Schedule of Study Visits and Evaluations **(Table 10-3)**. This spreadsheet will allow the investigator to calculate the number of times that each research-related activity is done for each subject and to include the appropriate numbers for all subjects in the protocol budget.

To develop this spreadsheet:

- Review the Protocol
- List all potential cost items
- Evaluate standard of care versus research-related test and procedures
- For multiyear studies, budget for each year (1st, 2nd, 3rd, etc.)

Study Drugs and Devices

Study Drugs

For sponsored research involving the use of an investigational drug, performed under an Investigational New Drug (IND) application, the sponsor, whether a pharmaceutical company or NIH, will supply the drug. For investigator-initiated research using an investigational drug or an approved drug for an investigational application, it is usually possible to arrange to have the drug company supply the drug for the research.

In research comparing approved drugs for approved uses, the subject's insurance or other third-party payer may cover the cost of the drug.

If the investigator is using a drug that is not available through a pharmaceutical company, the budget will need to include the costs of either compounding the drug or obtaining the drug from a consistent source throughout the course of the protocol.

TABLE **10-3** | Example of Schedule of Visits and Evaluations

Visits	1 (screen)	2 (baseline)	3	4	5	6	7	8	9	10
Weeks (from baseline)	−2 to −1	0	1	2	4	6	8	9	10	11
Visit window (±days)		Within 28 d	4	4	4	4	4	4	4	4
Study drug periods (drug kit dispensing)		A	B	C	D	E	F	G	H	
	Screening	Treatment period				Withdrawal period				
Informed consent	X									
Demographic data	X									
Diagnostic assessments: GAD (DSM-IV), MINI	X	X								
Ratings: HAM-A, CGI-S, MADRS, PWC, work and productivity, SDS, and WAT	X	X	X	X	X	X	X	X	X	X
Height	X									
Weight	X							X		X
T, P, R, BP	X	X	X	X	X	X	X	X	X	X
EKG	X							X		X
Physical exam	X							X		X
Safety lab 1	X							X		X
Safety lab 2						X				
Adverse events	X	X	X	X	X	X	X	X	X	X
Serious adverse events	X	X	X	X	X	X	X	X	X	X
Drug accountability			X	X	X	X	X	X	X	X
Concomitant medication	X	X	X	X	X	X	X	X	X	X

Study Devices

If research using a device is conducted under an Investigational Device Exemption (IDE), the sponsor provides the device for use in the protocol. Of course, if the investigator holds the IDE, the device would be a cost item for the budget. If a procedure is necessary for the placement of the device, this would also be considered investigational and included in the research budget.

Many device manufacturers will work with the FDA to obtain a classification for a new device (A, B, or C) based on technology that is the same or similar to a device that is already FDA approved. Research protocols using these devices, although still considered investigational research, will not include supplying the device, but rather will expect the investigator to bill the subject's insurance or third-party payer for the device and any expenses associated with it. The investigator will need to assure that the subject's insurance will pay these costs, either through a precertification process or by obtaining a coverage letter from the carrier (i.e., Medicare or Medicaid), and that the payment will cover the costs.

As with drugs, research involving the comparison of two approved devices is usually covered by a subject's insurance or other third-party payer.

Diagnostic Tests and Procedures

Research protocols can include diagnostic tests and procedures across the entire spectrum of available services and technologies. Some research is designed to test the accuracy or usefulness of new diagnostic tools or to compare new assays or procedures to existing ones.

General guidance on the costs of diagnostic tests and procedures is provided here. The investigator will need to carefully review the protocol to assure that accurate numbers are used to calculate cost. For example, a magnetic resonance scan is an expensive procedure. If the investigator forgets to include one at 3 months to assess changes in a tumor to determine response to a study drug, the budget overage could easily mount into thousands of dollars.

Some diagnostic tests and procedures also require professional interpretation. This will be charged by the physician (pathologist, radiologist, cardiologist, etc.) who performs the interpretation and will be in addition to the technical fee charged to perform the test.

As mentioned previously, for NIH-funded research, a vendor cannot charge more than Medicare will pay, so there may be a tiered pricing scale with a lower rate for NIH protocols and higher rates for industry-sponsored research. In preparing the budget, the investigator will need to obtain prices for each diagnostic test or procedure included in the protocol. For multiyear studies, it will be important to ask if these prices will remain the same throughout the course of the study, or if there will be annual adjustments.

Laboratory

Clinical Laboratory Tests

In most protocols, many clinical labs are required at screening to assure that the appropriate subjects are identified for enrollment in the study. For multicenter, sponsored research, the sponsor has usually made arrangements with a central laboratory to perform these tests. However, there may be a charge to have laboratory kits prepared for shipment.

Most investigators will have access to clinical laboratory services for investigator-initiated protocols. This may be a hospital laboratory or a commercial laboratory. The investigator will need to obtain a price list of the tests that the study will require. Often labs have a fee schedule based on the funding source for the research.

Pharmacological Testing

For the specialized testing that is necessary in the early phases of drug trials, the sponsor will make arrangements to any pharmacokinetic, pharmacodynamic, or pharmacogenomic testing. For the investigator who is developing and conducting this type of research, if his/her institution does not provide these services, these tests can be quite expensive. The investigator will need to analyze the study design carefully to assure that these tests are done as often as needed to answer the study questions, but not too frequently. (*Note*: Medicare does not have pricing for this type of laboratory testing, so there is no prescribed limit on charges.)

Genetic Testing

If a protocol includes genetic testing, or if the purpose of the research is to investigate the genetic basis of a disease or condition, the sponsor will make arrangements for this testing. For investigator-initiated research, this type of testing is usually done in the investigator's laboratory or other affiliated facility. There may or may not be direct costs associated with these tests.

Other Types of Laboratory Tests

Research involving blood and tissue banking, Genome-Wide Assay Studies (GWAS), human embryonic stem cells (hESC), or fetal tissue specimens are usually conducted at academic medical centers that have the infrastructure to support the collection, storage, and testing for these specialized protocols. The investigator will need to obtain cost figures for each of these activities. There may also be additional approvals necessary for this research and costs associated with submitting and obtaining approval.

Imaging

After clinical laboratory tests, imaging procedures are the most common diagnostic tests used in clinical research to identify appropriate subjects, obtain baseline information, and track the subject's response to the research. While simple x-rays may be relatively inexpensive, more complex computerized tomography (CT) scans, magnetic resonance imaging (MRI), and other advanced imaging procedures can be very expensive, especially if the procedure involves the use of contrast material or requires preparation prior to the test and/or observation afterwards. Research using emerging technologies (7 Tesla MRI, PET scans, etc.) will incur high costs.

The investigator will need to analyze the study design carefully to assure that these tests are done as often as needed to answer the study questions, but not too frequently. Costs will include not only the cost of the imaging test, but also any supplies, medications, and services that are not included in the basic cost, as well as interpretation fees (the professional component). Facilities have different policies on this pricing, and the investigator will need to assure that he/she has to total cost for budgeting purposes.

Some device studies are performed using interventional imaging procedures. For these protocols, which are usually industry sponsored, the investigator will need to assure cost coverage for both the device and the procedure, either by the sponsor or by subjects' third-party payers.

Cardiology

As with imaging, cardiology tests and procedures range from relatively inexpensive (EKG) to very costly (coronary imaging, balloon/stent procedures). As explained in the "Imaging" section, the investigator will need to obtain a complete list of all costs associated with the procedure.

Ancillary Costs

Operating Room, Anesthesia, Postanesthesia Recovery

Although often billed as hourly charges, most facilities are able to provide a composite fee for most surgical procedures, since this is how most payers process these charges. There should be a fee schedule for NIH-funded research and industry-sponsored protocols. However, if a protocol involves only part of the procedure (additional operating room time, only the anesthesia service, a study drug given in PACU), the investigator will need to work with the facility to obtain a cost figure for the research-related activity.

Observation Room Time

For most procedures, necessary observation room time postprocedure is included in the cost of the procedure. However, if participation in research includes observation, the facility can provide an hourly rate or fee schedule that the investigator can use to budget the costs.

Questionnaires, Evaluations, and Ratings

Many research protocols include the use of various questionnaires, evaluations, and ratings to provide baseline information and evaluate the subject's response to the study intervention. It is important for the investigator to use validated instruments for these assessments, whether the instrument is used in standard care (quality of life assessments, symptom evaluation questionnaires, pain scales) or is usually used only for research purposes (psychiatric evaluations and ratings, clinical global impression).

There are costs associated with the use of these instruments, which may include licensing fees, training and testing of research staff who will administer the assessment (to assure interrater reliability), and the services of a specialist consultant, if needed, to interpret results.

Payment for Subjects

Consideration of payments to subjects for participation in research is a complex process for investigators. If there is no payment, or the payment is not commensurate with risk, it may be difficult to enroll and retain subjects. If the payment is too high, there could be the appearance of coercion. Of course, if the sponsor will not allow these costs in the protocol budget, the issue is moot.

Compensation

To be clear, compensation is payment to subjects for their expenses associated with participation in the research. Will costs for travel, meals, parking, or child care be compensated? While meal or parking vouchers may be quite inexpensive, compensation for air travel and hotel costs are not. The investigator will need to consider the subject population and availability of funding in determining what costs can be reimbursed.

Compensation is not considered income for tax purposes. The investigator may be able to have a simple system to pay subjects for out-of-pocket expenses (a petty cash fund, vouchers, bus passes) that can save the costs of administering an account and issuing checks to subjects.

Incentive

Incentive payments are payments made to subjects for their participation in the research. The risk profile of the research, as well as any "burden of research" for the subject (frequency of visits, number of blood draws, pain or discomfort, etc.) should be considered in determining the appropriate incentive payments. In some institutions, an hourly rate is used to calculate incentive, while others use a more flexible study-by-study approach.

Incentive payments may be different (within the same protocol) based on the time, procedures, or inconvenience of the activities included in the visit. For example, if a subject must fast before a visit, have an intravenous line inserted, consume a glucose-containing beverage, and stay in the research center for 6 hours, this type of visit would support a higher incentive than one in which the subject just comes in for adverse event monitoring and to pick up a supply of study drug. However, the investigator must assure that incentive payments are not coercive, either to persuade subjects to participate in the research or to remain in the research when they would prefer to withdraw. Incentive schedules weighted to the final visits of a protocol are usually cited as examples of coercion.

Incentive payments are considered income for the subject, and payments must be calculated with appropriate withholdings. In general, the institution's Accounting Department (or similar) has procedures in place to set up an account for the research and issue payments (checks) to subjects with appropriate deductions. There may be a charge for this service, if it is not covered under the Facilities and Administration fee.

Other Types of Payment

For some protocols, there is neither compensation nor payment, but rather the sponsor is paying for a treatment or procedure that would otherwise be standard care or elective (as with cosmetic procedures) in order to collect data on a study drug, device, or intervention. The investigator will need to consider whether to include this type of cost in the protocol budget (if the funding agency will permit this) and whether the amount is commensurate with the risk profile of the study.

BUDGET MANAGEMENT AND MONITORING

Investigators must create a careful balance in the management and monitoring of protocol budgets. Budget deficits create problems including unpaid bills, loss of staff, and inability to complete the protocol, not to mention the impact on the investigator's relationship and credibility with the institution's administration. Excess funds also create problems: the funding source may require repayment of unspent money, or the institution may funnel the overage into a general fund before all data analysis activities have been completed.

Budget Management

Once again, the investigator will need to create a spreadsheet. The spreadsheet should detail the amounts budgeted for each of the research-related activities, payments with dates received, and calculations to assure that costs are adequately covered.

Upfront Payment

Research spending tends to be somewhat front-loaded, that is, the investigator incurs significant costs while preparing to begin the protocol. Many of these costs were previously described in the first sections of this chapter. Historically, industry sponsors would provide an initial payment (usually $5,000 to $10,000 or a percentage of the total budget) to offset these expenses. However, in the current environment, it is rare for an investigator to receive funds before the first subject is enrolled. NIH cooperative group protocols do not provide initial funding prior to enrollment. For grant-funded research, the grant may be fully funded upon receipt of IRB approval, depending on the payment source.

In summary, the investigator will need to assure that he has adequate resources and infrastructure to conduct all preliminary activities, including hiring of any additional staff, preparation of grant submissions and regulatory documents, obtaining cost figures and doing the budget, etc. prior to receiving initial payment.

Payments During the Conduct of the Research

Other than grant-funded research, most protocols base payment on enrollment of subjects and completion of Case Report Forms (CRFs). The more quickly an investigator can accomplish these activities, the sooner the payment stream will commence.

Screening/Screen Failures

For most protocols, the Screening Visit is the most expensive visit in the study schedule. Further, not all subjects who are screened will meet the inclusion and exclusion criteria to be enrolled in the study. The investigator will need to discuss with the sponsor the payment arrangements during the screening phase of the research. Will monitoring visits be conducted more frequently to facilitate collection of CRFs? Will the sponsor pay for the costs of screening for subjects who are unable to enroll in the research? Sometimes a sponsor will not provide full payment for screen failures, but will provide a percentage payment.

Payment upon Completion and Collection of Case Report Forms

In the environment of hard copy CRFs in triplicate, CRFs may be either mailed in to the sponsor or taken by the monitor upon completion of the monitoring visit. In either case, to maximize timely payment, it behooves the investigator to complete CRFs as soon as possible after subject visits are done, and to get monitor's comments and corrections addressed in time to have the pages pulled at the same visit.

Electronic CRFs also need to be completed as soon as possible. The software contains edits that provide prompts for data correction as pages are done, then the investigator (or member of the team) transmits the completed forms to the sponsor. Assure that there is a clear understanding about payment for these electronic forms. Will payment be sent as soon as pages are completed, or will further edits be sent prior to payment?

Final Payment

The investigator needs to assure that the study is adequately funded from initial activities through the final processes of data analysis. Sponsored research, whether industry or

NIH, usually has a provision for a final payment upon completion of all research-related activities and submission of all data as well as the return of study drug, study materials, and any equipment.

For grant-funded research, the investigator needs to assure that the budget will cover the costs until the end of the study, even if that is only a percentage of salary for final completion.

Budget Monitoring

Use of a spreadsheet as described above provides the best continuing resource for monitoring of the protocol budget. During the initial days and weeks of a study, when screening and frequent study visits are generating significant cost, the investigator (or designated member of the research team) will need to enter information timely, monitor weekly, postpayments promptly, and, in the case of sponsored research, work with the sponsor to assure that payments are sent and posted so that bills can be paid.

As the study moves forward, visits usually become less frequent, and costs are reduced. For multiyear protocols, the investigator will need to analyze staffing needs and other cost items as funding decreases.

Leveraging Resources

It's all about saving money. And there are some ways that an investigator can save money in the development and conduct of a clinical research protocol.

First, consider the standard of care for the disease or condition that is being studied. If laboratory tests, imaging procedures, or other diagnostic testing are done as standard care, the results can be collected for research purposes (with appropriate informed consent). The investigator needs to consider the time frame, that is, how recent must the results be to be valid for the purposes of his/her study? Is 1 month acceptable? Is 3 months too long? If most of the data required for screening can be collected from the subject's medical record, this can be a significant cost saving for the investigator. And if standard care schedules for repeat testing will provide sufficient data to answer the research questions, this will not only save money for the investigator but also save the subject the time, inconvenience, and discomfort of repeating the tests. Of course, the subject needs to be informed that his third-party payer will be billed for these tests and procedures.

Second, consider how often data must be collected, both to answer the research questions and to monitor subjects' safety. While visits may be frequent in the early part of the protocol (daily, weekly), visit intervals are typically extended as the study moves forward. However, it may be possible to collect some data by telephone contact or (secure) e-mail. Subjects can be asked about any new symptoms or adverse events, and some questionnaires, evaluations, and ratings can be done effectively over the telephone or in an electronic format. Consider whether visit intervals can be extended with the use of these interim contacts.

Third, make use of all available resources at the hospital, urban, or academic medical center or other institution. Many facilities now have a Research Department that provides research staff (nurses, coordinators, assistants) and services to clinical investigators. These may be done on a fee-for-service basis, allowing the investigator to pay for only those services that he needs, or, in some instances, the services may be covered under an institutional grant and provided free of charge to the investigator. Services may include preparation of regulatory documents, conducting study visits, completion of CRFs, conducting study-specific tests and procedures, and working with the sponsor and sponsor's representatives. In addition, some medical centers have dedicated inpatient and outpatient facilities available to investigators for the conduct of research-related activities. These fully staffed and equipped units can provide investigators with a convenient and economical resource for the conduct of clinical research protocols.

BIBLIOGRAPHY

1. Matula MA. Evaluating a protocol budget. In: Gallin JI, Ognibene FP, eds. *Principles and Practice of Clinical Research*. Burlington, MA: Academic Press; 2002.
2. Fine J, Albertsen PC. Budget development and staffing. In: Penson DF, Wei JT, eds. *Clinical Research for Surgeons*. Totowa, NJ: Humana Press Inc.; 2006.
3. Miskin BM, Neuer A. Budgeting. *How to Grow Your Investigative Site*. Boston, MA: CenterWatch; 2002.
4. Ginsberg D. Grants, budgeting and contracts. *Becoming a Successful Clinical Research Investigator*. Boston, MA: CenterWatch; 2005: 90–94.
5. Canfield D. Research budgeting. In: Schuster DP, Powers WJ, eds. *Translational and Experimental Clinical Research*. Philadelphia, PA: Lippincott Williams & Wilkins; 2005.
6. Reif-Lehrer L. *Grant Application Writer's Handbook*. Boston, MA: Jones and Bartlett Publishers, Inc.; 2004.

CHAPTER 11

Understanding Food and Drug Administration (FDA) Regulatory Requirements for Investigational New Drug Applications (IND) for Sponsor-Investigators

M. E. Blair Holbein, PhD

INTRODUCTION

Clinical investigators initiating a drug study invoke a number of specific regulatory requirements beyond those mandated for protection of human subjects in clinical trials (1). These regulatory requirements for drug studies address the safety and efficacy issues unique to the use of pharmaceuticals in the clinical research setting. The United States Food and Drug Administration (FDA) is charged with the regulation of most drugs in addition to other products. This extends to regulatory authority over clinical research utilizing these agents. Therefore, in order to conduct drug studies an investigator must comply with FDA requirements. Failing to meet the FDA's regulations can have legal and financial implications for the individuals conducting the research as well as the institutions associated with the research activities.

An initial part of the regulatory process involved for investigational drugs is notifying the FDA that a pharmaceutical agent will be used in an experimental way. This notification is called an "Investigational New Drug Application" (IND) (2). For drug trials conducted by the pharmaceutical industry or other commercial sponsors, individuals highly trained and expert in meeting the regulations address the regulatory requirements. However, for individual investigators who are not as familiar with the requirements and regulations, filing an IND can be intimidating and may be perceived as an impediment to conducting drug studies. It is interesting to note that the majority of IND submissions are noncommercial (3). Thus, individual clinical investigators frequently meet the regulatory requirements necessary to conduct investigational drug studies. This chapter is intended to address the simplest scenario in which an individual investigator initiates and conducts a drug study that requires filing and maintaining an IND with the FDA. Additionally, for the sake of simplicity, this review primarily addresses regulatory requirements for studies conducted at a single site. **Figure 11-1** depicts the IND application process for a Sponsor-Investigator.

THE REGULATORY ENVIRONMENT AND FDA ROLE

The FDA is an agency in the United States Department of Health & Human Services charged with assuring the safety, efficacy, and security of human as well as veterinary drugs in addition to other areas of regulatory authority. The agency is also responsible for facilitating advances in medications. The FDA is a large and rather complex federal agency with a number of centers, divisions, and offices. There are central offices in the Washington Metropolitan Area, numerous regional offices in the United States, and a small number of international offices. For the purposes of regulatory supervision of investigational drugs in human clinical trials, the centers primarily involved are the Center for Drug Evaluation and Research (CDER), Center for Devices and Radiological Health (CDRH), and the Center for Biologics Evaluation and Research (CBER). Within these centers are offices with regulatory, functional, or therapeutic focus. Most pharmaceutical drug products, both synthetic and biologic, fall under the regulatory supervision of CDER, including the majority of drug studies. CBER regulates biological and related products including blood, vaccines, allergenics, tissues, and cellular and gene therapies so only a small number of specialized drug studies would come under CBER jurisdiction (4). The FDA website publishes comprehensive organizational charts with the names and contact information for officials (4–6).

The primary set of federal laws establishing FDA authority as well as codification of the regulations is the Federal Food, Drug, and Cosmetic Act. The specific section of these laws covering an IND is in Part 312 of the Code of Federal Regulations (CFR). There are also other parts of the Federal Code that impact the conduct of clinical studies using

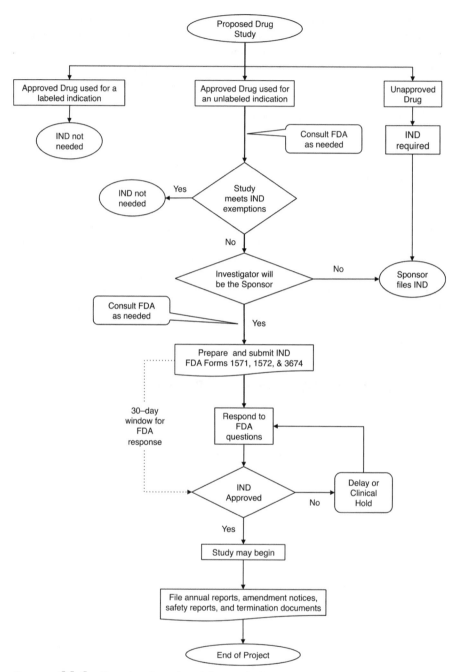

FIGURE 11-1   Flow chart for a clinical drug study that may require an investigational new drug (IND) application for an Sponsor-Investigator.

T A B L E **11-1** | Federal Regulations that Apply to the IND
Application Process

Code of federal regulations title 21 food and drugs

21CFR part 312	Investigational new drug application

Subparts and Sections discussed in text

312.2	Applicability (Exemptions listed in (b))
312.23	IND Content and Format
312.30	Protocol amendments (Reporting requirements)
312.31	Information amendments (Reporting requirements)
312.32	IND Safety reports (Reporting requirements)
312.33	Annual reports (Reporting requirements)
312.38	Withdrawal of an IND
312.42	Clinical holds and requests for modification
312.44	Termination
312.45	Inactive status
312.50	Responsibilities of sponsors
312.60	General Responsibilities of Investigators
312.61	Control of the Investigational Drug
312.62	Investigator Recordkeeping and Record Retention
312.64	Investigator Reports
312.66	Assurance of IRB Review
312.68	Inspection of Investigator's Records and Reports
312.69	Handling of Controlled Substances
312.70	Disqualification of a Clinical Investigator

Other relevant regulations

21CFR Part 314	INDA and NDA Applications for FDA Approval to Market a New Drug (New Drug Approval)
21CFR Part 316	Orphan Drugs
21CFR Part 50	Protection of Human Subjects
21CFR Part 56	Institutional Review Boards
21CFR Part 201	Drug Labeling
21CFR Part 54	Financial Disclosure by Clinical Investigators

IND, Investigational New Drug; NDA, New Drug Application; IRB, Institutional Review Board;
FDA, Food and Drug Administration.

pharmaceutical products. **Table 11-1** lists the more important sections relevant to individual investigators. All of these regulations are readily accessible at the FDA website in a searchable format (7). Finally, federal law dictates that in order for a drug to be transported or distributed across state lines it must have an "approved marketing application." Since drugs to be used in most clinical trials will be shipped across state lines the sponsor must seek an exemption from that legal requirement. The name "Notice of Claimed Investigational Exemption for a New Drug" refers to this exemption, but the more commonly used term is an "IND."

The stated purpose of an IND is "to ensure that subjects will not face undue risk of harm" in a clinical investigation that involves the use of a drug (8). Hence, in order to authorize a drug study in humans, the FDA requires sufficient information to assess the safety of the intended research study. The IND is the mechanism by which by the Investigator or Sponsor provides the requisite information to obtain authorization to administer an investigational agent to human subjects (or an approved drug used for a new indication or a new population of patients). All studies that use a drug not approved for marketing by the FDA will always require an IND. By a rather broad set of definitions for a "new drug" (9), all studies using not only new molecular entities or unapproved pharmaceuticals but also approved drugs used in unapproved indications, or in new formulations, or in new dosages, or in a patient population that would be put at increased risk, require an IND. However, under specific criteria, an exemption from this IND requirement may be met.

For regulatory purposes, clinical investigations involving drugs are initiated by a "Sponsor" who takes responsibility for the conduct of the study. This term applies to a number of different entities. A "Sponsor" can be an individual, a commercial entity such as a pharmaceutical company, an organization, or governmental agency. Sponsors may conduct large multicenter trials with unapproved drugs in the anticipation of submitting the results of such investigations in support of a New Drug Application or a change in the official labeling for an approved drug. IND applications for studies of this nature require a comprehensive dossier of information including animal studies, pharmacokinetic analyses, toxicology studies, and manufacturing information (CFR 312.23). A description of this type of complex commercial submission is beyond the intended scope of this chapter.

The FDA defines an "Investigator" to be the "individual who actually conducts a clinical investigation (i.e., under whose immediate direction the drug is administered or dispensed to a subject)" (2). Investigators may conduct clinical studies for a Sponsor. But, individual investigators, who initiate and conduct a clinical study as well as being directly accountable for the administration or dispensing of the investigational drug, are designated as a "Sponsor-Investigator" by the FDA. Clinical investigators at academic medical centers who are initiating clinical studies with a lawfully marketed drug to be used in a patient population or indication not within the official labeling often fit within this designation. Unlike a commercial sponsor initiating studies with an unapproved drug, often at multiple sites, a "Sponsor-Investigator" conducting an investigation at a single site will have a substantially less complicated filing requirement. The Sponsor-Investigator obtaining the IND would then be the "Holder" of the IND and thus would be responsible for the associated regulatory requirements. If the study is to be conducted at multiple sites or at multiple centers, there is still only a single entity responsible for interacting with the FDA.

WHEN IS AN IND NOT NEEDED FOR STUDIES INVOLVING MARKETED DRUGS?

Clinical trials that use an FDA-approved drug within the approved labeling do not need an IND. The use of a placebo does not require an IND if the investigation does not otherwise require submission of an IND. However, clinical investigations initiated by Sponsor-Investigators frequently make use of FDA-approved drugs in populations or indications not addressed in the approved labeling. Clearly such studies have a markedly different risk profile than a Phase I or II study with a new molecular entity. Correspondingly, the FDA has a mechanism to "bypass" filing an IND if specific exemption criteria are met that address the safety of the proposed study as well as stated limits on the noncommercial intent of the study. The exemption criteria only apply to studies using marketed pharmaceuticals commercially available in the United States. These criteria are listed in CFR 312.2(b). Importantly, all studies must also be approved by an Institutional Review Board (IRB) and informed consent procedures must be met as set forth in 21 CFR 50 and 56 in addition to meeting the exemption criteria. Note that studies involving an "exception from informed consent" all require an IND and cannot claim an exemption under these provisions.

For Sponsor-Investigators initiating a study with an approved drug, the exemption that most directly relates to safety issues is CFR 312.2(b)(iii). This criterion addresses whether the study "significantly increases the risks (or decreases the acceptability of the risks) associated with the use of the drug product" specifically regarding a route of administration, dosage level, dosage form, new proportions, or use in a patient population, or any other relevant study aspect that affects safety of drug use. For example, an investigator could make a case for an exemption for a study utilizing a drug in a disease entity not in the approved labeling, but reasonably supported by the underlying pharmacology with the provision that there are no anticipated increases in the risk of adverse effects from the drug for the study population.

The "noncommercial" context of the exemptions assures that the results will not be used to support a change in labeling for a new indication or a significant change in the advertising for the product. Such studies are typically undertaken by a pharmaceutical or device manufacturing company or other commercial entity. Analogously there must be a compliance with the requirements that the study does not amount to a commercial distribution or marketing of a new drug. The provisions do allow for charging the subject for the drug under narrow specified circumstances, however. Notably, FDA has issued additional guidance for exemption from IND for drugs used to treat cancer (10). Further provisions are made allowing exceptions for studies involving in vitro diagnostic biological products, blood grouping serum, reagent red blood cells, and antihuman globulin.

If a study does not meet the exemption criteria, then an IND may be required. If the Sponsor-Investigator has any question whether the study meets the exemption criteria, it is usually appropriate to contact the FDA to clarify the regulatory requirements. Likewise, the local IRB may also be able to help the investigator determine if the criteria for safety are adequately addressed in the study so as to avoid the need for an IND. If it is not clear whether or not an IND is required, contacting the FDA for clarification or discussion with the IRB can save a significant amount of time and effort. The organizational charts for CDER can be used to guide the initial phone contact. A Project Manager in the relevant division can provide significant help in addressing not only exemption requirements, but also in the IND application process, as well. Note that the FDA will not accept an application or review a study that is exempt under the stated provisions.

INVESTIGATIONAL NEW DRUG APPLICATION

There are different categories and types of IND. For individual Sponsor-Investigators the IND will be categorized as a "Research IND." The other category is "Commercial IND." The FDA categorizes IND applications as "Commercial" if the sponsor is either a corporate entity or one of the institutes of the National Institutes of Health (NIH) or if it is clear that the drug may be eventually commercialized. The FDA has issued numerous Guidances regarding filing an IND. The vast majority (80%) of the Guidances are addressed to Industry (i.e., commercial) (11).

Within the stated categories are a number of other designations. An "Investigator IND" is a Research IND submitted by an investigator who initiates and conducts the study including the immediate supervision of the use of the study drug. This would typify the studies conducted by Sponsor-Investigators. Additional IND types include an "Emergency IND" that allows the FDA to authorize use of an experimental drug in emergency situations that do not allow time for filing an IND or for patients who do not have access to the drug under protocol. Similarly, the "Treatment IND" allows access for subjects in serious or life-threatening situations to experimental drugs that have shown promise in early clinical testing but prior to final FDA review. Lastly, an "Exploratory IND" is conducted early in Phase I studies of an agent. These studies involve limited human exposure and are designed without therapeutic intent (screening, microdosing, etc.) and are preliminary to conducting more descriptive traditional safety and tolerance studies and allow for greater flexibility in the drug development process (9).

Additionally, for antimicrobial products the FDA has a consultation program to facilitate communications between the Sponsor and the FDA prior to filing an IND involving the treatment of bacterial, fungal, and viral infections, opportunistic infections, emerging infections (including naturally emerging diseases and potential biothreat agents), topical microbicides directed at prevention of HIV transmission, and transplant rejection (12).

GENERAL PRINCIPLES

The general scheme for an IND includes providing information in general areas: Animal Pharmacology and Toxicology Studies, Manufacturing Information, and Clinical Protocols and Investigator Information. The intent is to provide information to the FDA to allow a review that assures the safety of participants. For Sponsor-Investigators, typically, the IND will not require the same extensive information including preclinical studies or manufacturing and process information as would be required for a commercial sponsor applying for an IND for a yet unapproved drug, especially early in its development. To an extent, this is because the studies conducted by Sponsor-Investigators usually use FDA-approved pharmaceuticals with an established clinical profile. Note too that a Sponsor-Investigator has responsibilities as both a Sponsor and Investigator.

IND GUIDANCE AND PLANNING

For commercial sponsors, drug development is a far more complex and involved process compared to that for Sponsor-Investigators. Analogously, the pre-IND process is more formalized and often entails scheduled meetings or teleconferences. For Sponsor-Investigator, most questions are typically less complicated. Nonetheless, individual investigators can and should make use of the agency resources. The FDA website has downloadable forms, descriptions of the IND application process, and listings of guidance on the completion of the forms and clerical requirements (13). The FDA has issued Guidance that addresses the IND submission process specifically for Sponsor-Investigators (14). Extensive information for Sponsors to guide Preclinical and Phase I studies and Pre-IND consultations is also listed. The FDA makes contact information for both CDER and CBER officials available on the FDA website. Questions about the IND process can be directed to the appropriate Office or Division, generally by telephone or email.

FDA FORM 1571

The Investigational New Drug Application, FDA Form 1571, provides the structure to present the information about the proposed research. By definition, "the Sponsor is the person who takes responsibility for and initiates a clinical investigation. The sponsor may be a pharmaceutical company, a private or academic organization, or an individual." Hence, an individual investigator who initiates (e.g., designs, and obtains funding) and conducts (e.g., directly responsible for administration or dispensing the investigational drug) a research study meets the criteria of a Sponsor-Investigator (14). Note especially, even if a pharmaceutical company will supply drugs or placebos, the individual investigator is still the named Sponsor. For Sponsor-Investigators parts of the information required on the 1571 overlap with and are covered by the FDA Form 1572.

Form 1571 is used by all applicants, commercial as well as clinical investigators, and there are several sections that do not apply to a Sponsor-Investigator. Likewise, since the IND from the Sponsor-Investigator involves the use of an FDA-approved drug, several responses in the 1571 are abbreviated, amended, or even omitted compared to a pharmaceutical industry sponsor. Specifically, no designation is needed for Phase of Study (Section 8), IND Number (Section 6) is left blank with initial application, Contract Research Organization (Section 13) should be marked "no," and contact information for Sponsor representative (Sections 18 and 19) is left blank. Finally, the serial number is "0000" with the initial application (Section 10). Subsequent IND amendments increase the serial number by 1 in the order of submission.

Since the study drug is a commercially available product, the information required by the FDA will be modified for a Sponsor-Investigator compared to an industrial sponsor. If the marketed drug will be used "without modification to its approved packaging," the 1571 should contain the trade name, generic name, dosage form, strength, and lot number. Drug Master Files (21 CFR 314.42), Product License Applications (21 CFR Part 601), or the Investigator's Brochure are generally not required.

If a product will be provided in a nonapproved form, then manufacturing and controls information, pharmacology and toxicology data, or data from prior human studies will be required unless that information has previously been submitted to FDA. If this is the case, then a means for the FDA to reference the previous information will be needed. Typically this can be done via a letter from the original sponsor that authorizes access and includes the file identification (IND/DMF/NDA) number. If the dosage form will be modified by the investigator, then manufacturing and controls information, pharmacology and toxicology data, or data from prior human studies may be required. Discussion with the FDA can help clarify what additional information is needed.

The section entitled "Contents of the Application" (Section 12) is likewise abbreviated for most Sponsor-Investigator submissions. For this section, items 2, 3, and 4 (Table of Contents, Introductory Statement, and General Investigational Plan, respectively) may be addressed in the cover letter. The information detail is not dissimilar to information required by most local Institutional Review Boards. Projects utilizing commercially available pharmaceutical products that will be used without modification can be adequately described by reference to their standard identifiers (names, dosage forms, and strength). The "Environmental Assessment" (Section 7) can be addressed with a categorical exclusion statement, "I claim categorical exclusion (under 21 CFR 25.31[e]) for the study(ies) under this IND. To my knowledge, no extraordinary circumstances exist." However, if the pharmaceutical agent is modified in any way, additional information may be required. All manufacturing (or compounding) information should be submitted. Likewise, if the agent has the potential for drug dependence or abuse, if it is radioactive, or if it will be used in pediatric studies, additional information may be needed. A more detailed description of the information required is contained in 21 CFR 312.23.

For all forms in the IND application, the Sponsor-Investigator is the single person responsible for the conduct, progress, review, and evaluation of safety associated with the trial. It is important to provide complete and consistent contact information for all forms and correspondence. The correspondence address and the telephone number listed should also indicate the most effective contact information for the individual Sponsor-Investigator, including a daytime phone number.

There are slight differences in completing and submitting the 1571 for CBER than for CDER (15). Due to the highly specialized nature of CBER studies, investigators should consult CBER directly for guidance.

FDA FORM 1572

This form comprises the "Statement of Investigator." The information requested regarding the Investigator's qualifications and contact information can often be met by an academic curriculum vita noting on the form that the information is contained in the attachment. Note also that for Sponsor-Investigator sections of the FDA Form 1572 satisfy the information requirements for specific sections of the FDA Form 1571. The IND requirement to supply information regarding qualifications of each investigator (16) who will participate in the study could technically be met by submitting the information with the 1571; it is far simpler to have each investigator complete a separate FDA Form 1572.

FDA FORM 3674

The IND application must be accompanied by a certification that the requirements of section 402(j) of the PHS Act have been met. U.S. Public Law 110-85 (Food and Drug Administration Amendments Act of 2007 or FDAAA), Title VIII, Section 801 requires registration of "applicable clinical trials" (17). All controlled clinical investigations that use a drug regulated by the FDA must be registered with the exception of Phase I studies. The intent of the legislation requiring that applicable clinical studies be registered is to ensure that the public has access to information about certain clinical trials that are being conducted, including access and results. This registration process is done via filing trial information with the Protocol Registration System (PRS) of clinical trials run by the United States National Library of Medicine (NLM) at the National Institutes of Health (NIH) (18). Form 3674 certification requires the appropriate ClinicalTrials.gov identifiers (NCT numbers) that are obtained from registration. The FDA has issued draft guidance on the certification process (19).

For a Sponsor-Investigator filing an IND, the responsibility for registration rests with the investigator. For most Sponsor-Investigators the institution with the regulatory oversight for the conduct of the study is probably already a registered research entity with a registration account and the investigator will not need to create a separate registration account.

ADDITIONAL INFORMATION FOR MULTICENTER TRIALS

Some Sponsor-Investigator–initiated trials will be conducted at more than one site. This includes trials at sites all within the regulatory oversight of a single IRB as well as multiple sites each under the purview of the separate affiliated institutional boards. It is the responsibility of the Sponsor-Investigator to compile all the associated required information for each participating site into a single IND application. This includes information regarding the facilities, laboratories, each separate IRB or a central IRB (if one is used), all investigators, drug accountability, and preparation (if applicable). Much of the required information will fall under Section 12 of the FDA Form 1571. While each investigator will have a separate FDA Form 1572, these are compiled and submitted under a single FDA Form 1571. Likewise, all correspondence with the FDA occurs with the Sponsor-Investigator who files the FDA Form 1571.

SUBMITTING AN IND

A cover letter should accompany the IND submission. Include identification of the Sponsor-Investigator, a clear indication that this is an initial IND submission, and assure that the contact information is clear and complete. Since this is the initial IND submission, there is no IND number. Each sequential correspondence regarding an IND should carry a sequential identifying serial number, which in this initial submission would be "0000." Clearly indicate the title of the study. Take care that the contact information exactly matches that in 1571 and 1572 to avoid any delays in communications. Since this process is time-sensitive, delays due to communication errors can have significant consequences. Send the submission to the attention of the Division that oversees the therapeutic area for the study drug. If there has been a discussion with an individual at CDER or CBER, they may direct the submission to a specific recipient. The IND should be submitted in triplicate, an original and two copies. No special binders or packaging is required. **Table 11-2** lists the submission addresses.

TABLE **11-2** | Submission Addresses

IND submissions to CDER for a Drug:	Food and Drug Administration Center for Drug Evaluation and Research Central Document Room 5901-B Ammendale Road Beltsville, MD 20705-1266
IND submissions to CDER for a Therapeutic Biological Product:	Food and Drug Administration Center for Drug Evaluation and Research Therapeutic Biological Products Document Room 5901-B Ammendale Road Beltsville, MD 20705-1266
IND submissions to CBER for a Biological Product:	Center for Biologics Evaluation and Research HFM-99, Room 200N 1401 Rockville Pike Rockville, MD 20852-1448

FOLLOWING RECEIPT OF IND BY THE FDA

The IND will be routed to the appropriate division for review. A letter of acknowledgement will be sent to the Sponsor-Investigator. This letter provides the assigned IND number, date received, and the name and telephone number of the FDA Project Manager to whom questions about the application and further correspondence should be directed. The IND becomes effective 30 days after the stated FDA receipt date unless the FDA sends notification otherwise. The FDA generally does not send a letter notifying the Sponsor-Investigator of approval. Studies may begin after the 30-day interval, if the FDA does not notify the investigator otherwise. If the FDA requests further information or clarification, the 30-day window is not affected unless the FDA gives an indication that the study is placed on a Complete or Partial Clinical Hold. A Partial Hold will allow a specific part of the study to begin while the other part cannot be started. A "Clinical Hold" explicitly means that the study may not begin.

RESPONDING TO A CLINICAL HOLD

A "Clinical Hold" occurs when the FDA contacts the Sponsor-Investigator and indicates that the study cannot start pending resolution of questions or concerns. The specific questions that the agency has are conveyed to the investigator, typically by phone followed by a detailed letter. Upon receipt of the list of FDA concerns, the Sponsor-Investigator should respond to the issues cited in the letter in their entirety. The cover letter that accompanies the response should clearly indicate the response with a heading "Clinical Hold Complete Response." Likewise, the accompanying FDA Form 1571 should indicate by serial number and checkbox that it is a response to a Clinical Hold. The "clock" on the review process does not begin until all issues have been addressed and the responses have been received and acknowledged by the FDA.

The FDA should reply within 30 days of the receipt of the complete response from the Sponsor-Investigator. The agency will issue a letter that either lifts the Clinical Hold (the study may proceed) or places the study on partial hold (specific restrictions) or that the study continues on hold pending resolution of continuing questions. Until the FDA indicates that a hold has been removed, a study must not proceed.

REGULATORY REQUIREMENTS FOR AN IND DURING STUDY AND AT COMPLETION

Submission of an IND begins the regulatory process under which a study progresses. There are on-going obligations that the Sponsor-Investigator agrees to with the signature of the FDA Form 1571. In brief, the Sponsor-Investigator agrees to keep the IND current, to notify the FDA about any safety issues, to file annual reports, and to notify the FDA when the study ends for any reason. Any amendment to the IND must be filed with the FDA.

Protocol Amendments (21 CFR 312.30)

Provisions in this section allow for the filing of a new protocol, changes to protocol, or the addition of a new investigator. Changes can include any increase or decrease in drug exposure by way of dose or duration, a change in the subject population inclusion or exclusion, or a change in monitoring for safety. The IRB with oversight responsibility must likewise be notified and give approval. The amended protocols must be submitted prior to implementation with the exception of a protocol change intended to eliminate an apparent immediate hazard to subjects. In this case, the IRB is notified in accordance to regulations and the FDA subsequently notified.

Information Amendments (21 CFR 312.31)

Similar to amendments in the research protocol, changes in the essential information regarding the IND that are not within other reports are added via an "Information Amendment." This can include changes in toxicology, chemistry, or other technical information. All amendments should be clearly labeled as to the contents (e.g., "Information Amendment: Pharmacology-Toxicology"). These amendments should not be issued more frequently than 30-day intervals.

Safety Reports (21 CFR 312.32)

Sponsor-Investigators are responsible for investigating all safety concerns brought to their attention. They must notify the FDA, all participating investigators, and the local IRB of any adverse experience associated with the use of the drug that is both serious and unexpected in a written IND Safety Report. This equally applies to any finding that suggests a significant risk for human subjects. The timeframe for reporting is no later than 15 calendar days after the sponsor's initial receipt of the information. The report should be made via FDA Form 3500A (MedWatch) or in a narrative format. The report should be clearly labeled "IND Safety Report." The Sponsor-Investigator is responsible for analyzing the significance of the report in context of other safety reports.

In the case of either death or life-threatening experience associated with the study drug, notification of the FDA must be made no later than 7 calendar days after the Sponsor-Investigator's initial receipt of the information. This should be done either by telephone report or by facsimile transmission. The local IRB should likewise be informed.

Annual Reports (21 CFR 312.33)

Annual reports must be filed by the Sponsor-Investigator. The filing deadline is within 60 days of annual date of the IND. If there are multiple protocols under a single IND, each should be identified by title and have a summary report. The investigator should include the status of each study still in progress and each study completed during the previous year. The progress of enrollment should be tallied including total number of subjects planned, number entered to date (by age, gender, and race), the number of subjects whose participation in the study was completed as planned, and the number who dropped out of the study for any reason. If the study has been completed or if interim results are known, a brief report of results should be included. A summary of all IND safety reports submitted during the past year should be included. A summary of any significant changes in the pharmacology, toxicology, or technical information should be included. Lastly, the plan for the coming year should be stated.

WITHDRAWAL, TERMINATION, AND INACTIVATION

A sponsor may withdraw an IND at any time. The FDA and all investigators should be notified and all drug stocks accounted for. If the withdrawal is for safety reasons, the notification must provide a report of the reasons. In this case, the reviewing IRB must also receive notification. When a study ends, the Sponsor-Investigator must notify the FDA.

The FDA may terminate an IND. This is usually done in cooperation with the Sponsor, but may be unilateral. The Sponsor is allowed a response to an FDA-initiated termination, but the timeframe is quite limited.

A study may be placed on "Inactive status" by the Sponsor or the FDA. This may be due to a number of reasons such as delays in implementation, insufficient enrollment, failure to file annual reports, or failure to respond to FDA inquiries. An IND that remains in inactive status for 5 or more years may be terminated.

MONITORING RESPONSIBILITIES FOR SPONSOR-INVESTIGATORS

Monitoring of the study is an on-going responsibility. The regulations explicitly charge the Sponsor-Investigator with accountability. Sponsors must monitor and assure that human subjects are adequately protected, that all reported clinical data are accurate and complete, and that the conduct of the trial is in compliance with the protocol and regulations. Unique to drug studies is the added responsibility for drug accountability. Investigators must also correct any problems that occur during the study or terminate the study and notify their IRB, the FDA, and other investigators.

ADDITIONAL INFORMATION FOR MULTICENTER TRIALS

As with submission of an IND for a multicenter trial, the Sponsor-Investigator is accountable for all interim and terminal reporting. All amendments, annual reports, changes in investigators (FDA Form 1572), and safety reports are compiled by and filed with the FDA by the Sponsor-Investigator. Equally, it is the responsibility of the Sponsor-Investigator to assure that each participating site is fully informed about all modifications including any FDA actions or correspondence. Importantly, the Sponsor-Investigator is also accountable for assuring that each site is working from the most recent amended protocol, the respective regulatory documents are submitted to the respective IRBs, and all regulatory requirements for the study are met across all sites.

CONCLUSION

Meeting the regulatory requirements for conducting drug studies is an essential part of doing clinical research. Filing and maintaining an IND may seem intimidating. But, a Sponsor-Investigator, working with the FDA, can meet the regulatory obligations and can proceed with their research study with minimal delay. The FDA makes it easy to contact the officers who are responsible for handling the IND. The guidance for filing the necessary documents is comprehensive and readily available from the FDA website. Filing and maintaining an IND should not be regarded as an impediment to doing clinical drug research.

ACKNOWLEDGMENT

This work is supported in part by NIH CTSA Grant UL1 RR024982.

REFERENCES

1. Federal Food, Drug, and Cosmetic Act.
2. CFR Title 21 Part 312 "Investigational New Drug Application"
3. CDER ORIGINAL INDs RECEIVED CALENDAR YEARS 1986–2008. Available at: http://www.fda.gov/downloads/Drugs/DevelopmentApprovalProcess/HowDrugsare DevelopedandApproved/DrugandBiologicApprovalReports/UCM165257.pdf. Accessed June 16, 2009.
4. Center for Biologics Evaluation and Research Organization. May 28, 2009. Available at: http://www.fda.gov/AboutFDA/CentersOffices/OrganizationCharts/ucm135943.htm. Accessed June 16, 2009.
5. CDER Center for Drug Evaluation and Research Organization. May 28, 2009. Available at: http://www.fda.gov/AboutFDA/CentersOffices/OrganizationCharts/ucm135674.htm. Accessed June 16, 2009.

6. Department of Health and Human Services Food and Drug Administration Center for Drug Evaluation and Research. Available at: http://www.fda.gov/downloads/AboutFDA/CentersOffices/OrganizationCharts/UCM144011.pdf. Accessed June 16, 2009.

7. CFR—Code of Federal Regulations Title 21. April 1, 2009. Available at http://www.accessdata.fda.gov/scripts/cdrh/cfdocs/cfCFR/CFRSearch.cfm. Accessed May 12, 2010.

8. Guidance for Industry, Investigators, and Reviewers, Exploratory IND Studies. January 12, 2006. Available at: http://www.fda.gov/downloads/Drugs/GuidanceComplianceRegulatory Information/Guidances/UCM078933.pdf. Accessed June 16, 2009.

9. Code of Federal Regulations Title 21 Part 310. "New Drugs."

10. Guidance for Industry. IND Exemptions for Studies of Lawfully Marketed Drug or Biological Products for the Treatment of Cancer. Available at: http://www.fda.gov/downloads/Drugs/GuidanceComplianceRegulatoryInformation/Guidances/UCM071717.pdf. Accessed June 16, 2009.

11. FDA/CBER - Investigational New Drug (IND) Guidances. April 30, 2009. Available at: http://www.fda.gov/BiologicsBloodVaccines/DevelopmentApprovalProcess/InvestigationalNew DrugINDorDeviceExemptionIDEProcess/ucm094297.htm. Accessed June 16, 2009.

12. Division of Antiviral Products - ODE IV Pre-IND Consultation Program. June 16, 2009. Available at: http://www.fda.gov/Drugs/DevelopmentApprovalProcess/HowDrugsareDevelopedand Approved/ApprovalApplications/InvestigationalNewDrugINDApplication/Overview/ucm077776.htm. Accessed June 16, 2009.

13. Investigational New Drug (IND) Application. June 2, 2009. Available at: http://www.fda.gov/Drugs/DevelopmentApprovalProcess/HowDrugsareDevelopedandApproved/Approval Applications/InvestigationalNewDrugINDApplication/default.htm. Accessed June 16, 2009.

14. Information for Sponsor-Investigators Submitting Investigational New Drug Applications (INDs). April 30, 2009. Available at: http://www.fda.gov/Drugs/DevelopmentApprovalProcess/SmallBusinessAssistance/ucm071098.htm. Accessed June 16, 2009.

15. Investigational New Drug (IND) or Device Exemption (IDE) Process (CBER). June 15, 2009. Available at: http://www.fda.gov/BiologicsBloodVaccines/DevelopmentApprovalProcess/InvestigationalNewDrugINDorDeviceExemptionIDEProcess/default.htm, Accessed June 16, 2009.

16. 21 CFR 312.23(a) (6)(b)

17. U.S. Public Law 110-85 (Food and Drug Administration Amendments Act of 2007), Title VIII, Section 801.

18. Protocol Registration System Information. Available at https://register.clinicaltrials.gov/. Accessed May 14, 2009.

19. Guidance for Sponsors, Industry, Researchers, Investigators, and Food and Drug Administration Staff. Certifications To Accompany Drug, Biological Product, and Device Applications/Submissions: Compliance with Section 402(j) of The Public Health Service Act, Added By Title VIII of The Food and Drug Administration Amendments Act of 2007. June 8, 2009. Available at: http://www.fda.gov/RegulatoryInformation/Guidances/ucm125335.htm. Accessed June 16, 2009.

Collecting Data

Deanna S. Adams, RN

INTRODUCTION

After writing the protocol in consultation with a biostatistician, the next step is to consider the data needed to (1) answer the study questions (achieve objectives) and (2) assure compliance with the requirements of the federal regulations, Human Subject Protection (HSP), and Good Clinical Practice (GCP).

In this chapter, information will be provided on the collection, recording, validation, and protection of the data required for a research protocol.

DATA COLLECTION

Definitions

What is de-identified? Throughout this chapter, the term "de-identified" will be used repeatedly. It is important to have a clear understanding of this term as it pertains to the collection of research data on human subject participants. De-identified means "the information is recorded by the investigator in such a manner that subjects cannot be identified, directly or through identifiers linked to the subjects." [45 CFR 46.101 (b) (4)]

RESEARCH ETHICS: PITFALLS & PRESCRIPTIONS

While the current definitions of "identifiers" and "de-identified" data hold as of 2010, clinical investigators should expect and look out for new requirements in protecting the privacy of clinical data. As the comprehensive clinical databases described in Chapter 4 proliferate in academic medical centers, data profiling using extensive clinical, genomic, proteonomic, biobanking, and other indicators will permit identification of unique patients and research subjects, even when protecting the current HIPAA identifiers. This means that new regulations and ethical guidelines will emerge, as the clinical-scientific landscape changes and investigators using these research resources should be aware and be ready to respond accordingly.

Greely HT. The uneasy ethical and legal underpinnings of large-scale genomic biobanks. *Annu Rev Genomics Hum Genet*. 2007;8:343–364.

What is an identifier? Identifiers are defined in the Health Insurance Portability and Accountability Act (HIPAA) Privacy Rule [45 CFR 164.501, 164.508, 164.512(i)] **(Table 12-1)**.

Exempt Research

Some protocols consist solely of the collection of de-identified retrospective data from medical records, the analysis of de-identified blood or tissue samples (e.g., laboratory or surgical waste) that would otherwise be wasted. These types of studies (and others as described in the regulations) are not considered to be research on human subjects as defined by the Office for Human Research Protections (OHRP). Consult the OHRP website for additional information: http://www.hhs.gov/ohrp/humansubjects/guidance/45cfr46.htm#46.101.

Institutional Review Boards (IRBs) have policies and procedures in place to further define research considered exempt from review. The investigator should consult with the IRB to assure compliance with any local requirements.

Expedited Research

"*Minimal risk* means that the probability and magnitude of harm or discomfort anticipated in the research are not greater in and of themselves than those ordinarily encountered in daily life or during the performance of routine physical or psychological examinations or tests" (45 CFR 46).

For protocols that present the potential for no more than Minimal Risk to subjects, OHRP defines categories of Expedited Research (45 CFR 46.110) **(Table 12-1)**.

If the proposed research appears to meet the criteria of no more than Minimal Risk and to fit into one of the nine categories described above, the investigator should consult the IRB regarding procedures for submission and approval of Expedited research. Expedited review is often appropriate for certain types of databases and blood and tissue banking protocols.

Obtaining Preliminary Data

As described in this section, preliminary data may refer to retrospective data collected from existing medical records or databases, or information obtained prior to consent to identify potential subjects for a research protocol.

TABLE **12-1** | Identifiers

1. Names
2. Social security numbers
3. Telephone numbers
4. All geographic subdivisions smaller than a State, including street address, city, county, precinct, zip code (there are some provisos)
5. All elements of dates (except year) for dates directly related to an individual, including birth date, admission date, discharge date, date of death, and all ages over 89
6. Fax numbers
7. Electronic mail addresses
8. Medical record numbers
9. Health plan beneficiary numbers
10. Certificate/license numbers
11. Account numbers
12. Vehicle identifiers and serial numbers, including license plate numbers
13. Device identifiers and serial numbers
14. Web Universal Resource Locators (URLs)
15. Internet Protocol (IP) address numbers
16. Biometric identifiers, including finger and voice prints
17. Full face photographic images and any comparable images
18. Any other unique identifying number, characteristic, or code (note this does not mean the unique code assigned by the investigator to code the research data). A limited data set is described as health information that excludes the direct identifiers listed above, except that may include city, state, ZIP Code, elements of date, and other numbers, characteristics, or codes not listed as direct identifiers. A data use agreement is needed to obtain satisfactory assurances that the recipient of the limited data set will use or disclose the PHI in the data set only for specified purposes.

Some protocols consist solely of the collection of retrospective data for analysis. This type of research is inexpensive, easy to accomplish, and can usually be done very quickly (in a matter of days or weeks). The data collected and analyzed from this type of study can be used to inform the development of future protocols.

Examples could include

1. A retrospective comparison of different surgical procedures, different devices, or different treatment regimens for a particular disease or condition. Data might include the diagnosis and procedure codes, length of stay, laboratory reports, cost, etc.
2. A demographic analysis on the number of patients admitted to a hospital during a specific time period with a particular diagnosis. Again, data might also include information on gender, ethnicity, age, length of stay, etc.
3. Longitudinal analysis of disease treatment and experience over a specified period of time (for example, 5 years). Data might include episodes of care, complications, medications, laboratory reports, etc.

4. Establishment of a database for a particular disease or condition, including the collection of contact information, date of diagnosis, medications and treatments, etc. Often these databases are used not only for data analysis, but also for recruitment for participation in future research.

While de-identified information collected in examples (1) and (2) might qualify as Exempt research, the identifiers necessary in examples (3) and (4) would fall under the Expedited category. Some IRB's may require an initial Full Board Review for establishment of a database.

The HIPAA Waiver or "What You Can Get Without Getting Consent"

Preliminary data may also be obtained to identify potential subjects who may be eligible to enroll in a research project. HIPAA allows an investigator to obtain a limited amount of information prior to consent if the following criteria are met:

- The Protected Health Information (PHI) use or disclosure involves no more than a minimal risk to the privacy of individuals based on at least the presence of (1) an adequate plan presented to the IRB or Privacy Board to protect PHI identifiers from improper use and disclosure; (2) an adequate plan to destroy those identifiers at the earliest opportunity, consistent with the research, absent a health or research justification for retaining the identifiers or if retention is otherwise required by law; and (3) adequate written assurances that the PHI will not be reused or disclosed to any other person or entity except (a) as required by law, (b) for authorized oversight of the research study, or (c) for other research for which the use or disclosure of the PHI is permitted by the Privacy Rule.
- The research could not practicably be conducted without the requested waiver or alteration.
- The research could not practicably be conducted without access to and use of the PHI.

This is called a Waiver or Alteration of the HIPAA Authorization.

If potential subjects are not patients of the investigator, a HIPAA Waiver allows the investigator to obtain PHI

- from the medical record or
- during an initial telephone contact or scheduled visit

The HIPAA Waiver should only contain the minimal necessary information to determine eligibility. This may include

- Contact Information (name, address, telephone)
- Demographics (age, gender, ethnicity)
- Medical History
- Current Medications
- From the medical record:
  - Billing Information (admitting/discharge diagnoses, length of stay, total charges, etc.)
  - Most Recent Physical Reports
  - Surgical and Pathology Reports
  - Results of Diagnostic Testing (lab, imaging, cardiology, etc.)
  - Medications and Treatments

- Physicians' Orders and Progress Notes
- Discharge Summary

The investigator should be aware that PHI obtained under a HIPAA Waiver must be either de-identified or destroyed within a reasonable period of time for subjects who do not enroll (consent) in the research. The investigator will need to consult with his/her Institutional Review Board or facility administration to obtain specific guidance and time limits.

For example, an investigator may want to study diabetic peripheral neuropathy. As a beginning, the investigator could use the diagnosis code (249.6) to obtain a limited data set from the medical records of the institution. The data collected could include name, date of birth, medical record number, dates of admission and discharge, length of stay, medications, surgical procedures, therapies, etc. After preliminary analysis, the data must be de-identified **(Table 12-1)**. This could be done by assigning each patient a subject number, using initials instead of a name, using age instead of date of birth, and removing the medical record number and any dates. The investigator could then use the information to inform a prospective study; the investigator would know how many subjects he/she could enroll within a given timeframe, average lengths of stay, standard care treatment at the institution, common complications, etc.

Blood and Tissue Banking/Repositories

As previously described, the use of de-identified blood or tissue samples that would otherwise be laboratory or surgical waste is considered Exempt research.

However, establishment of blood or tissue repositories that use identified samples, samples associated with PHI, or samples to analyze familial patterns are not "Exempt." These activities require IRB review and approval and are subject to specific regulations and guidance from OHRP and the Food and Drug Administration (FDA). The National Heart, Lung, and Blood Institute (NHLBI) issued the following guidance based on current regulations **(Table 12-2)**.

T A B L E   **12-2** | Blood and Tissue Banking Repositories

Operating Principles

1. The concept of a tissue repository may include two kinds of samples: (a) those collected with the expressed purpose of distribution to investigators and (b) those collected by individual investigators and not originally intended to be shared with others, but which are subsequently shared as part of a repository. Any collection that contains specimens that are potentially identifiable and are distributed to someone other than the investigator (or in the case of a multiinvestigator study, other than any of the identified investigators) making the collection, regardless of the original intent, may be considered to be a repository.

2. Any identifiable tissue (included coded tissue) that is collected requires IRB review at the site of collection (even if different from the site of the repository) and, under most circumstances, written informed consent from the subject. Where possible, informed consent should include information about the repository and the conditions under which tissues will be shared (e.g., see NCI sample consent above).

(continued)

T A B L E   **12-2** | **Blood and Tissue Banking Repositories** *(continued)*

3. Any tissue repository that distributes materials requires an IRB, convened under an OPRR-approved assurance, that lays out the conditions under which the tissue will be shared. These conditions must consider the privacy of the individuals from whom the tissue came, what the informed consent permitted, and the intent of the person to whom the tissue is sent.

4. A committee, established under the repository IRB's guidelines, must evaluate each request for samples to see if the request is consistent with the IRB's conditions for sharing samples and with the original informed consent. The IRB at the repository institution may choose to perform this committee's functions itself.

5. The recipient of the tissue samples must abide by the conditions specified by the repository IRB. This need not, but may, include review and approval by an IRB at the recipient's organization.

6. Exemptions to the need for IRB review and informed consent may be made if the tissue samples are truly unable to be tied to an individual. Samples that are coded do not qualify for an exemption, as someone has the key to the code.

7. Even if the samples do not formally constitute a repository, IRB approval at the institution where the samples are stored is required if the collector/distributor is an NIH employee or if the storage is for the purpose of sharing and that sharing is supported by funds from the Department of Health and Human Services. The need for IRB approval in other situations depends on the institution's OPRR-approved Assurance.

    (1) Clinical studies of drugs and medical devices only when condition (a) or (b) is met.

        (a) Research on drugs for which an investigational new drug application (21 CFR Part 312) is not required. (Note: Research on marketed drugs that significantly increases the risks or decreases the acceptability of the risks associated with the use of the product is not eligible for expedited review.)

        (b) Research on medical devices for which (i) an investigational device exemption application (21 CFR Part 812) is not required or (ii) the medical device is cleared/approved for marketing and the medical device is being used in accordance with its cleared/approved labeling.

    (2) Collection of blood samples by finger stick, heel stick, ear stick, or venipuncture as follows:

        (a) from healthy, nonpregnant adults who weigh at least 110 pounds. For these subjects, the amounts drawn may not exceed 550 ml in an 8-week period and collection may not occur more frequently than 2 times per week; or

        (b) from other adults and children (2), considering the age, weight, and health of the subjects, the collection procedure, the amount of blood to be collected, and the frequency with which it will be collected. For these subjects, the amount drawn may not exceed the lesser of 50 ml or 3 ml per kg in an 8-week period and collection may not occur more frequently than two times per week.

    (3) Prospective collection of biological specimens for research purposes by noninvasive means. Examples:

        (a) hair and nail clippings in a nondisfiguring manner

        (b) deciduous teeth at time of exfoliation or if routine patient care indicates a need for extraction;

(continued)

T A B L E **12-2** | *(continued)*

(c) permanent teeth if routine patient care indicates a need for extraction;

(d) excreta and external secretions (including sweat);

(e) uncannulated saliva collected either in an unstimulated fashion or stimulated by chewing gumbase or wax or by applying a dilute citric solution to the tongue;

(f) placenta removed at delivery;

(g) amniotic fluid obtained at the time of rupture of the membrane prior to or during labor;

(h) supra- and subgingival dental plaque and calculus, provided the collection procedure is not more invasive than routine prophylactic scaling of the teeth and the process is accomplished in accordance with accepted prophylactic techniques;

(i) mucosal and skin cells collected by buccal scraping or swab, skin swab, or mouth washings;

(j) sputum collected after saline mist nebulization.

(4) Collection of data through noninvasive procedures (not involving general anesthesia or sedation) routinely employed in clinical practice, excluding procedures involving X-rays or microwaves. Where medical devices are employed, they must be cleared/approved for marketing. (Studies intended to evaluate the safety and effectiveness of the medical device are not generally eligible for expedited review, including studies of cleared medical devices for new indications.) Examples:

(a) physical sensors that are applied either to the surface of the body or at a distance and do not involve input of significant amounts of energy into the subject or an invasion of the subject's privacy;

(b) weighing or testing sensory acuity;

(c) magnetic resonance imaging;

(d) electrocardiography, electroencephalography, thermography, detection of naturally occurring radioactivity, electroretinography, ultrasound, diagnostic infrared imaging, Doppler blood flow, and echocardiography;

(e) moderate exercise, muscular strength testing, body composition assessment, and flexibility testing where appropriate given the age, weight, and health of the individual.

(5) Research involving materials (data, documents, records, or specimens) that have been collected or will be collected solely for nonresearch purposes (such as medical treatment or diagnosis). (Note: Some research in this category may be exempt from the HHS regulations for the protection of human subjects. 45 CFR 46.101(b)(4). This listing refers only to research that is not exempt.)

(6) Collection of data from voice, video, digital, or image recordings made for research purposes.

(7) Research on individual or group characteristics or behavior (including, but not limited to, research on perception, cognition, motivation, identity, language, communication, cultural beliefs or practices, and social behavior) or research employing survey, interview, oral history, focus group, program evaluation, human factors

(continued)

T A B L E **12-2** | Blood and Tissue Banking Repositories *(continued)*

evaluation, or quality assurance methodologies. (Note: Some research in this category may be exempt from the HHS regulations for the protection of human subjects. 45 CFR 46.101(b)(2) and (b)(3). This listing refers only to research that is not exempt.)

(8) Continuing review of research previously approved by the convened IRB as follows:

    (a) where (i) the research is permanently closed to the enrollment of new subjects; (ii) all subjects have completed all research-related interventions; and (iii) the research remains active only for long-term follow-up of subjects; or

    (b) where no subjects have been enrolled and no additional risks have been identified; or

    (c) where the remaining research activities are limited to data analysis.

(9) Continuing review of research, not conducted under an investigational new drug application or investigational device exemption where categories two (2) through eight (8) do not apply but the IRB has determined and documented at a convened meeting that the research involves no greater than minimal risk and no additional risks have been identified.

Other NIH Institutes provide similar guidance for establishment and use of blood and tissue repositories. The Office for Protection of Research Risks provides a flow chart **(Table 12-3)**.

There are also special considerations and requirements for research involving human embryonic stem cells (hESC), fetal tissue specimens, and genome-wide assay studies (GWAS). Consult the appropriate NIH websites for regulations and guidance. Each local IRB will also have policies and procedures for these types of activities.

Data Collection During the Research

Screening

The Screening Visit is typically a lengthy visit beginning with the consent process and continuing through all activities, tests, and procedures required to determine whether or not a potential subject is appropriate for enrollment in the research protocol. (See **Table 12-4** for examples of screening activities.)

Document the consent process and review of the Inclusion and Exclusion Criteria in the source file to verify that the subject has met all requirements prior to beginning study procedures.

Study Visits and Research-Related Activities

In determining the frequency of study visits, the investigator should consider the data needed to answer the study questions and any identified safety concerns.

Visits may include

- Randomization
- Drug accountability and dispensing of study drug

T A B L E   **12-3** | Issues to Consider in the Research Use of Stored
                       Data or Tissues

Department of Health and Human Services, November 7, 1997

Human Tissue Repositories collect, store, and distribute human tissue materials for research purposes. Repository activities involve three components: (i) the **collectors** of tissue samples, (ii) the **repository** storage and data management center, and (iii) the **recipient** investigators.

- If supported by the Department of Health and Human Services (HHS), each component must satisfy certain **regulatory requirements**.

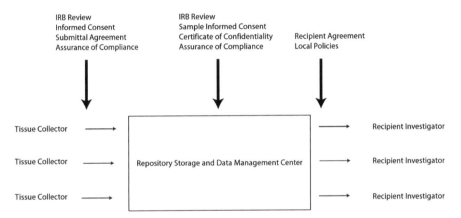

- Operation of the Repository and its data management center should be subject to **oversight by an Institutional Review Board (IRB)**. The IRB should review and approve a protocol specifying the conditions under which data and specimens may be accepted and shared and ensuring adequate provisions to protect the privacy of subjects and maintain the confidentiality of data. The IRB should also review and approve a sample collection protocol and informed consent document for distribution to tissue collectors and their local IRBs. A **Certificate of Confidentiality** should be obtained to protect confidentiality of repository specimens and data.

- Updating of baseline information
- Frequency of research-related procedures (lab, radiology procedures, questionnaires, evaluations and ratings, pharmacokinetic and pharmacodynamic testing, etc.)
- Monitoring for adverse events (2,3)
  - Subject report
  - Safety labs

Assure that the data gathered is sufficient to

- Meet the biostatistical requirements to evaluate the stated objectives of the research
- Evaluate and report relevant safety concerns

TABLE **12-4** | Screening Visit Activities, Tests, and Procedures

- Consent and HIPAA authorization
  - Special circumstances

Mental status examination or assessment of cognitive function – will the subject require a Legally Authorized Representative (LAR) for surrogate consent?
Blood alcohol level (BAL, i.e., breathalyzer) or urine drug screen (UDS) – if the subject is intoxicated, is consent valid?

- Baseline information (see previous information under Preliminary Data)
- Update H&P (recent events, psychiatric history, alcohol and/or drug use, HIV status, etc.)
- Current (concomitant) medications
- Vital signs
- Laboratory tests
  - CBC, chemistry, urinalysis
  - Pregnancy testing
- Study-specific (thyroid, lipid panel, HIV, Hepatitis, etc.)
- For clinical trials using a study drug: pharmacokinetics, pharmacodynamics, biomarkers
- Imaging (CT, MRI, X-ray)
- Electrocardiogram (EKG)
- Questionnaires, evaluations and ratings (diagnostic interviews, pain scales, symptom assessments, functional evaluations, psychiatric ratings, quality of life, etc.)

Follow-Up

Depending on the nature of the research, the investigator may need to include provisions for follow-up in the protocol. Some considerations include

- Monitoring of subjects' medical records for a defined period after participation in the research to collect data on continued care, hospital admissions, or other information pertinent to the subjects' responses to the research.
- Long-term follow-up (e.g., until disease progression or death) for protocols testing new drugs or treatment modalities. This is often seen in oncology research. Consider the frequency of data collection and whether this will be done through visits or telephone contact.
- Continued access to a study drug for subjects that have a positive response during the research and the data to be collected.

DATA RECORDING

Source Documents

By definition, source documents are the first place that information is recorded. This could be the medical record or source documents specific to the research protocol.

The Medical Record

The medical record, governed by numerous federal and state laws and regulations and monitored by various oversight agencies and commissions, remains the best source document for research. Data collected from the medical record is, by its nature, validated, verifiable, and retrievable. Whether in hard copy or electronic versions, the medical record contains a wealth of information (laboratory reports, radiology reports, lists of medications, etc.) that can assist the investigator in identifying potential subjects, and in screening and monitoring the subject's condition during participation in the research.

Medical record departments keep logs of the persons who request charts. Electronic systems maintain audit trails of persons who have accessed records. The investigator must assure that he/she (or any member of the research team) has the appropriate authorization in place in order to view and collect data from the medical record. (See previous information regarding HIPAA regulations on the access to and use of this information.)

At academic medical centers and hospitals, electronic medical records (EMRs) may provide software modules specifically designed for research. Consultation with Information Technology or Bioinformatics (if available) department staff can assist the investigator in utilizing these modules to capture the necessary data for a research project.

The Source File

In many cases, a medical record is not available, and the investigator must build a source file to capture essential data. Many sponsors provide source document templates based on the necessary data that must be acquired at each visit. If source documents need to be developed, the investigator can easily create a format using the schedule of visits and procedures. These visit notes should not contain personal identifiers but can be identified with initials or a subject number. Allow adequate space for a narrative note. The person completing this note should sign and date it. Some sponsors may also require the principal investigator to sign and date these notes to verify that he/she has reviewed the information (Appendix I and **Table 12-5**).

TABLE **12-5** | Guidance for Documentation in the Source File

1. Write legibly and neatly.
2. Black ink only (no pencil or colored pens).
3. No erasures, correction fluid (white out, liquid paper), or tape.
4. Make corrections one line striking through the error, write the corrected information, then initials and date.
5. Use only accepted abbreviations (medical, Standard English). Hint: When in doubt, write it out.
6. Any original information should be saved as source (i.e., a self-stick note with vital signs on it could be source).
7. Document all telephone contacts and attempts, with or pertinent to the subject.
8. Identify each source document with the subject's name, initials, or subject ID.
9. Save everything!

Special Topics

Innovative Approaches for Data Collection

In addition to traditional pen-and-paper methods and EMRs, investigators are utilizing emerging technologies to develop and implement new types of tools to collect research data. In Social, Behavioral, and Economic Research (SBER), computer surveys allow subjects to complete de-identified questionnaires that provide information on knowledge and behavior to answer research questions in areas as diverse as colon cancer and the impact of catastrophic events (hurricanes and earthquakes) (4–7).

Investigators are also using subject's personal electronic devices (cell phones, blackberries, etc.) to send real-time queries that provide valuable data regarding the subject's condition between scheduled visits.

Case Report Forms

Case Report Forms (CRFs) are the most familiar tool by which investigators record and communicate study data. Historically, these forms were provided in triplicate with an original to be archived by the sponsor and copies for data entry and the study binder.

In the current environment, electronic CRFs that incorporate auditing functions and data analysis capabilities are the preferred method for recording research data. Initiatives (and mandates) from NIH and FDA as well as improved software technology and the availability of Biomedical Informatics consultation for investigators have made electronic capability accessible to most investigators.

Electronic Data Collection and Reporting

In May 2007, the FDA published a useful guidance document, "Guidance for Industry – Computerized Systems Used in Clinical Investigations," that contains the agency's current thinking on electronic data collection and reporting. This document provides information on electronic source documents, data transmission, audit trails, and other issues pertinent to the conduct of clinical trials in an electronic environment. This document is available on the FDA website.

Biomedical Informatics

The expanding capabilities of Biomedical Informatics (or Bioinformatics) provide investigators with a toolbox of options:

- For the capture, management, and exchange of research data.
- To support the interrogation of EMRs for subject recruitment and involvement, as well as research-related hypothesis testing using biological and clinical data integrated from multiple sources.
- To support effective data management and analysis.

Depending on the nature of the research, software can be programmed for

- Scheduling and tracking appointments
- Tracking laboratory specimens
- Acquiring and validating a wide range of data types
- Monitoring and controlling study progress

- Generating management reports
- Reporting results to subjects
- Supporting family studies
- Long-term tracking of subjects' locations and health status
- Maintenance of database security and confidentiality

The research database may include multiple data types: survey results, clinical data, lab analysis results, genetic data, ECG/waveform data, and imaging data, and even microarray analysis of gene expression.

Academic medical centers often obtain federal funding to develop software for research applications that are then made available in the public domain. (Information here excerpted from the *Biomedical Informatics* section of the "North and Central Texas Clinical and Translational Science Initiative" grant written by Richard H. Scheuermann, Ph.D. Milton Packer, MD, Principal Investigator.)

DATA VALIDATION

The FDA has established standards for data collected in the course of a clinical trial, ". . . fundamental elements of data quality (e.g., attributable, legible, contemporaneous, original, and accurate). FDA's acceptance of data from clinical trials for decision-making purposes depends on FDA's ability to verify the quality and integrity of the data during FDA on-site inspections and audits" (21 CFR 312, 511.1(b), and 812). In brief, the data must be validated.

Training

The investigator is responsible for assuring that each member of the research team has been properly trained. Training and certification in HSP, HIPAA research regulations, and GCP are expected. For each protocol, team members will also require training in the study-specific procedures. Depending on the nature of the study, this may include

- Use of specific equipment (e.g., sphygmomanometer, EKG machine, and cups for urine drug screens)
- Accurate measurement of vital signs (blood pressure, temperature, pulse, respirations) (8)
- Procedures for drawing blood
- Processing of blood or tissue samples
- Potential risks of the study drug, device, or intervention
- Monitoring requirements based on potential risks
- Completion of questionnaires, evaluations, or ratings

Consistency

The investigator needs procedures in place to assure that study data are collected in a consistent manner. Put another way, the same thing should be done in the same way each time. As much as possible, the same equipment should be used each time a blood pressure or EKG is recorded. Study drug should be obtained from the same supplier each time or compounded by the same pharmacist. Interpretation of EKG's and radiology images should be done by the same radiologist.

For laboratory reports, the investigator should assure that all laboratory analyses are done in a lab certified by the College of American Pathologists (CAP) and operated in compliance with the Clinical Laboratory Improvement Amendments (CLIA). The laboratory will supply the investigator with normal ranges for all available tests. These ranges should be used by the investigator (and programmed into any software) to identify abnormal results.

For protocols that use questionnaires, evaluations, and ratings as data collection tools, the protocol should use only validated instruments. If the purpose of the research is to validate a new instrument, the investigator should make this clear, and the protocol should include the administration of validated tools against which the new tool will be compared.

All raters must be appropriately trained in the conduct and completion of these tools (9,10). For some instruments, a level of education or clinical experience may be required to assure valid results. As much as possible, it is preferable that the same rater conducts these sessions with the subject each time. If this is not possible, the investigator should perform and document both training and testing of all team members to assure inter-rater reliability.

For questionnaires, evaluations, and ratings as well as diaries, medication logs, and other data collection tools that are completed by the subject, the investigator needs to assure that the subject has received clear instructions (11,12). This includes instructing the subject in the proper method for correcting any mistakes that are made to avoid questions about the accuracy and validity of this data.

While subjective rating scales (visual analogue scales and Clinical Global Impression) may be useful to indicate a subject's response, data from these scales should not be the primary means to evaluate study objectives. When these ratings are completed by both the subject and the clinician, there are often significant differences.

Validation of Electronic Data

In the FDA Guidance referenced earlier, the agency places great emphasis on the programming of software to be used to collect record or transmit data from research protocols. "We recommend that you incorporate prompts, flags, or other help features into your computerized system to encourage consistent use of clinical terminology and to alert the user to data that are out of acceptable range." Fields need to be designed with appropriate ranges that will identify outlier values. Fields should not auto-populate. The system should create and maintain an audit trail for data corrections that includes the person, date (month/day/year), and time that each change was made.

DATA PROTECTION

For the protection of hard copy research documents that contain subject identifiers (consent) or protected information (source files), accepted methods are locked files in locked offices with access limited to members of the research team.

Similarly, research data stored on computers is password protected with access limited to members of the research team. The FDA further recommends that team members do not share passwords and that the computer will revert to an automatic screensaver and require password re-entry if time has elapsed since last use.

Use of portable devices, whether it is a laptop computer, personal digital assistant, zip or thumb drives, or other type of emerging technology, presents an array of problems in research. Loss or theft of these devices could result in the sharing of subjects' protected health information, a HIPAA violation. Data could be irretrievably lost. The investigator must consider carefully whether the convenience of these devices outweighs the potential risks of their use.

Software used for the collection, reporting, and/or transmission of research data requires safeguards at each point in the process. The FDA states, "Procedures and controls should be put in place to prevent the altering, browsing, querying, or reporting of data via external software applications that do not enter through the protective system software." Data transmitted off-site must also be protected through encryption.

Certificate of Confidentiality

If a protocol includes the collection of sensitive information that may have psychological, social, or economic risks for subjects, the investigator should consider obtaining a Certificate of Confidentiality. Examples of this type of information include, but are not limited to, genetic testing, HIV/AIDS, and psychiatric or substance abuse, especially in treatment-naïve subjects.

As explained by the National Institutes of Health (NIH), Certificates of Confidentiality are issued by the NIH to protect the privacy of research subjects by protecting investigators and institutions from being compelled to release information that could be used to identify subjects with a research project. Certificates of Confidentiality are issued to institutions or universities where the research is conducted. They allow the investigator and others who have access to research records to refuse to disclose identifying information in any civil, criminal, administrative, legislative, or other proceeding, whether at the federal, state, or local level.

Although access is restricted, medical records can be obtained by insurance companies, physicians, and others through a HIPAA Release of Information. The medical record can also be accessed as part of a legal proceeding upon issuance of a subpoena. If it is known that a subject is participating in a research protocol, a subpoena can also compel release of research records. If information in the research record is not otherwise discoverable (i.e., would not be in the subject's existing medical record), a Certificate of Confidentiality provides an extra layer of protection for the subject.

The NIH Institutes provide Certificates of Confidentiality based on the investigator's area of research. Information, contact persons, and applications can be found at http://grants.nih.gov/grants/policy/coc/

Note: A Certificate of Confidentiality does not protect the subject or relieve the investigator from mandated reporting requirements. Each state has regulations regarding reporting of infectious diseases as well as reporting abuse of children, the disabled, and the elderly. The investigator should access information from the state department of health regarding reporting requirements.

REFERENCES

1. Slieker FJ, Kompanje EJ, Murray GD, et al. SAPHIR and Pharmos TBI Investigators. Importance of screening logs in clinical trials for severe traumatic brain injury. *Neurosurgery*. 2008;62(6): 1321–1328; discussion 1328–1329.

2. Bibawy H, Cossu A, Cogan S, et al. Reporting of harms and adverse events in otolaryngology journals. *Otolaryngol Head Neck Surg*. 2009;140(2):241–244.

3. Coplan P, Chiacchierini L, Nikas A, et al. Development and evaluation of a standardized questionnaire for identifying adverse events in vaccine clinical trials. *Pharmacoepidemiol Drug Saf*. 2000;9(6):457–471.

4. Kauer SD, Reid SC, Sanci L, et al. Investigating the utility of mobile phones for collecting data about adolescent alcohol use and related mood, stress and coping behaviours: Lessons and recommendations. *Drug Alcohol Rev*. 2009;28(1):25–30.

5. Bidargaddi NP, Sarela A. Activity and heart rate-based measures for outpatient cardiac rehabilitation. *Methods Inf Med*. 2008;47(3):208–216.

6. Graham AL, Papandonatos GD. Reliability of internet- versus telephone-administered questionnaires in a diverse sample of smokers. *J Med Internet Res*. 2008;10(1):e8.

7. Rivera ML, Donnelly J, Parry BA, et al. Prospective, randomized evaluation of a personal digital assistant-based research tool in the emergency department. *BMC Med Inform Decis Mak*. 2008;8:3.

8. Lee J, Park D, Oh H, et al. Digital recording system of sphygmomanometry. *Blood Press Monit*. 2009;14(2):77–81.

9. Rosen J, Mulsant BH, Marino P, et al. Web-based training and interrater reliability testing for scoring the Hamilton Depression Rating Scale. *Psychiatry Res*. 2008;161(1):126–130. Epub 2008 Aug 30.

10. Thomas N, Unsworth B, Ferenczi EA, et al. Intraobserver variability in grading severity of repeated identical cases of mitral regurgitation. *Am Heart J*. 2008;156(6):1089–1094. Epub 2008 Oct 9.

11. Wolpin S, Berry D, Austin-Seymour M, et al. Acceptability of an Electronic Self-Report Assessment Program for patients with cancer. *Comput Inform Nurs*. 2008;26(6):332–338.

12. Trull TJ, Solhan MB, Tragesser SL, et al. Affective instability: measuring a core feature of borderline personality disorder with ecological momentary assessment. *J Abnorm Psychol*. 2008;117(3):647–661.

CHAPTER 13

Data and Safety Monitoring

Andrea M. Nassen, RN, MSN

INTRODUCTION

This chapter presents a synopsis of the role of data and safety monitoring in clinical trials. Data monitoring is the process of reviewing accumulated outcome data to optimize the continuing safety of current and future research subjects and to evaluate the validity and scientific merit of the trial. Practical information is provided to guide researchers in the formulation of meaningful Data and Safety Monitoring Plans (DSMPs) and, when indicated, the constitution of entities to monitor data and safety monitoring. Fundamentals addressed include definitions of these tools, the rationale for their requirement, and strategies for their development.

DATA AND SAFETY MONITORING PLANS

What Is a Data and Safety Monitoring Plan (DSMP)?

A DSMP is a description of systems and strategies set in place to guide the requisite oversight and monitoring of study conduct (1). The plan should commensurate with the nature

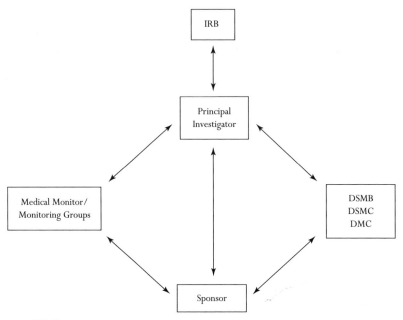

FIGURE **13-1**   Monitoring entities specified in the Data and Safety Monitoring Plan may fall anywhere along a continuum from monitoring by the Principal Investigator to monitoring by an independent Data and Safety Monitoring Board (DSMB)/Data and Safety Monitoring Committee (DSMC)/Data Monitoring Committee (DMC). Intermediary entities may include Medical Monitors or Monitoring Groups that may be established either by the Principal Investigator or the study Sponsor. Reporting relationships between and among entities tend to vary and require clarification prior to study initiation.

of the research study (i.e., biomedical or behavioral) and its size, scope, complexity, level of risk, and participant population. The plan should specify the person or entity responsible for oversight, the parameters to be assessed, the level and frequency of monitoring and reporting, and the methods to be utilized. Monitoring entities specified in the DSMP may fall anywhere along a continuum from monitoring by the Principal Investigator (PI) to monitoring by an independent Data and Safety Monitoring Board (DSMB)/Data and Safety Monitoring Committee (DSMC)/Data Monitoring Committee (DMC). Intermediary entities may include Medical Monitors or Monitoring Groups that may be established by the PI or by the study Sponsor (**Figure 13-1**). Reporting relationships between and among entities tend to vary and, thus, require clarification prior to study initiation.

Who Is Responsible for Data and Safety Monitoring?

The PI is primarily responsible for the safe and ethical conduct of human research, for study supervision and for the protection of the rights, safety, and welfare of research subjects. Additionally, the PI bears responsibility for the development of the DSMP, for designation of the monitoring entity, for submission of the DSMP to the Institutional Review Board (IRB) at the time of initial review, for compliance with the DSMP over the life of the protocol, and for reporting updates to the IRB at the time of continuing review and more frequently, as indicated. The DSMP should be developed prior to grant application (e.g., National Institute of Health, NIH) and protocol submission to the IRB and should be finalized prior to subject enrollment.

Why Is a DSMP Required?

There are two principal sets of regulations governing human subjects' research, those promulgated by the Food and Drug Administration (FDA) and those enforced by the Office of Human Research Protections (OHRP). The FDA regulates use of experimental drugs, devices, and biologics. Among OHRP's many activities are the drafting of policy guidance, development of educational programs and materials, regulatory oversight, and the provision of advice on ethical and regulatory issues in biomedical and behavioral research. Both agencies are within the Department of Health and Human Services (DHHS), the United States government's principal agency for protecting the health of all Americans and providing essential human services. The FDA's regulations are found at 21 Code of Federal Regulations (CFR), parts 50 and 56 (2). The policy guiding the protection of all human research subjects (regardless of whether or not FDA has jurisdiction) is found at 45 CFR Part 46/Protection of Human Subjects, Subpart A (1). The policy, commonly referred to as *The Common Rule*, states in section §46.111 that (1)

- Risks to subjects are minimized by using procedures which are consistent with sound research design and which do not unnecessarily expose subjects to risk;
- Risks to subjects are reasonable in relation to anticipated benefits, if any, to subjects, and the importance of the knowledge that may reasonably be expected to result;
- When appropriate, the research plan makes adequate provision for monitoring the data collected to ensure the safety of subjects; and
- When appropriate, there are adequate provisions to protect the privacy of subjects and to maintain the confidentiality of data.

Do All Studies Require a DSMP?

All interventional studies involving more than minimal risk must include a DSMP. Interventional research refers to any prospective study involving human subjects, which is designed to answer specific questions about the effects or impact of a particular biomedical or behavioral intervention (e.g., drugs, devices, treatments or procedures or behavioral or nutritional strategies) or to answer specific questions about human physiology. A study is considered to be more than minimal risk if the probability and magnitude of harm and/or discomfort anticipated in the research are greater than those ordinarily encountered in daily life or during the performance of routine physical or psychological examinations or tests (1,2). Some noninterventional studies requiring full board IRB review may also require a DSMP.

Over the years, several policy statements and guidance documents have been published describing which studies require a DSMP. The 1998 NIH Policy Statement communicated that data and safety monitoring is required for all types of clinical trials including Phase I (i.e., physiologic, toxicity, and dose-finding studies), Phase II (e.g., efficacy studies), and Phase III (i.e., efficacy, effectiveness, and comparative studies). In the 2000 Policy

Statement, investigators were required to submit a DSMP as part of the research plan for Phase I and II trials. Each NIH institute has a policy defining its institute-specific system for data and safety monitoring. Additional guidance is available from organizations such as the National Cancer Institute (NCI) and other agencies.

What Are the Essential Elements of a DSMP?

Although overall elements of a DSMP may vary, essential elements include

- Study risks (e.g., low, moderate, high)
- Type of data or events to be monitored including
  - Study accrual or enrollment
  - Experiences of study subjects
  - Study attrition including subject withdrawals and dropouts
  - Adverse events and unanticipated problems including the nature, severity, and frequency of events that might be expected and or possibly or likely related to the research
  - Protocol deviations and violations
  - Changes in risk/benefit
- Safety monitoring methods including the
  - Frequency of assessments of data or events
  - Persons and/or entities responsible for monitoring, reviewing, analyzing, and reporting data (e.g., principal investigator, research sponsor, coordinating or statistical center, medical monitor, and DSMB/DSMC/DMC)
  - Steps to protect the confidentiality of data collected
  - Steps to protect the privacy of subjects
  - Steps to minimize risks and discomforts to subjects
- Nature and frequency of interim analyses (i.e., the plans for reviewing safety and efficacy data) and the statistical tools to be utilized in the analysis
- Specific triggers or stopping rules dictating endpoints when some type of action is required (e.g., study alteration or termination). Studies may be stopped when there is greater than expected morbidity or mortality or when the experimental arm in a comparison study is shown to be better or worse statistically than the standard care arm.
- Rules for withdrawing participants from study intervention(s)
- Procedures and timetable for communicating adverse events and outcomes of reviews to the IRB, the study sponsor, and/or other indicated entity (e.g., NIH and FDA)

WHAT ARE APPROPRIATE MONITORING ENTITIES & METHODS?

Depending on the size, complexity, and inherent risk of the protocol, one or more individuals or groups may be described in the DSMP as bearing responsibility for data and safety monitoring. Options include but are not limited to the investigator, study staff, an independent monitor or expert, independent monitoring groups, or independent Data and Safety Monitoring Board. Boards are also referred to as Data and Safety Monitoring Committees (DSMCs) or Data Monitoring Committees (DMCs). These entities may be established by the

PI or the study sponsor (e.g., industry-sponsored trials). Regardless of other monitoring entities and methods in place, the PI is ultimately responsible for the onsite protection of human subjects, the safe and ethical conduct of research activities, and study oversight.

Investigator

For many studies, the PI will be the monitoring entity. This is appropriate when the study involves a small number of subjects, the study is conducted only at one site, and the range of possible study events that could have an important impact on the risks and benefits to research participants is narrow. In such cases, ongoing monitoring of events by the investigator and study staff and prompt reporting of adverse events and unanticipated problems to the IRB and FDA or others as appropriate may be adequate.

The issue of possible conflicts of interest must be taken into account, especially if the investigator assumes the role of the monitor. Use of an independent monitor or expert can address the need for an unbiased review. Independent review can be achieved through a range of solutions.

Independent Monitor or Expert

The investigator can enlist the assistance of a physician or other appropriate expert who is independent of the study and available real time to review study data and recommend appropriate actions regarding adverse events and other safety issues. The name and qualifications of the expert should be included in the DSMP submitted to the IRB at the time of initial review.

Independent Monitoring Committee

Monitoring Committees tend to be small groups comprised of several independent investigators and a biostatistician who review data from a particular study. The independent investigator may be recruited within an institution or from an outside institution.

Data Safety Monitoring Board (DSMB)/Data Safety Monitoring Committee (DSMC)/Data Monitoring Committee (DMC)

DSMBs, DSMCs, and DMCs are terms interchangeably used to describe formal groups specifically established to provide ongoing monitoring of data and subject safety throughout the life of a protocol. Their primary responsibility is to collect and analyze data to monitor for adverse events and other trends that would warrant modification or termination of the trial or notification of subjects about new information that might affect their willingness to continue in the trial. The group has a specific composition or membership and a specific charter or list of primary responsibilities including monitoring, reviewing, and reporting. Proceedings are guided by a chairperson, appointed prior to the first meeting, responsible for developing agendas, facilitating discussions, and compiling and submitting reports.

The group's composition usually consists of three or more multidisciplinary members with knowledge, talents, and experience in areas relevant to a particular research question. Areas of applicable expertise might include the surgical or medical specialty of interest, clinical trial methodology, biostatistics, bioethics, or population demographics. To minimize conflicts of interest, the committee should be independent of trial organizers and investigators.

A typical charter might include a table of contents; an introduction; primary responsibilities of the DSMB/DSMC/DMC; group membership, including members and conflicts of interest; timing and purpose of meetings, including the organizational meeting, early safety/trial integrity reviews, and formal interim efficacy analysis; procedures to ensure confidentiality; communication at closed sessions, open sessions, open and closed sessions, minutes of the meetings, and recommendations to the PI; statistical monitoring guidelines; and content of the DSMB's open and closed reports. Of note, there is a growing trend to create Institutional Data and Safety Monitoring Boards. Pools of biostatisticians, researchers, ethicists, clinicians, and scientists are compiled from which individual boards can be assembled and customized to meet investigators' needs. A template of a DSMP is included in Appendix J.

A DSMB/DSMC/DMC may be the most appropriate way to monitor data and safety for studies that involve

- Large study populations in which risk may be better assessed through statistical comparisons of treatment groups
- Multiple clinical sites where there is a need for investigators to submit reports of adverse events to a central reporting entity, such as a coordinating center or statistical center, responsible for preparing timely summary reports of adverse events for distribution among the clinical sites, and to the IRBs
- High-risk interventions in which death or severe disability is a major risk of research participation
- High expected rates of morbidity or mortality in the study population (e.g., natural history of disease or aging)
- High chance of early termination for reasons of safety, futility, or efficacy
- Blinded study treatment groups in which the validity and integrity of the study may be adversely affected by having an individual or group associated with the design and conduct of the study break the blind
- Randomized design
- Controlled trials with mortality or major morbidity as primary or secondary endpoints where increased morbidity or mortality may be better assessed through statistical comparisons among treatment groups.
- Vulnerable populations (e.g., pediatrics and geriatrics)
- Novel therapies (e.g., gene therapy and xenotransplantation)
- Conflicts of interest
- High public interest or public perception of risk
- NIH study at the discretion of the sponsoring Institute

External DSMBs are generally not needed for

- Single-site trials
- Single-arm trials
- Early phase trials
- Short-term trials of treatments to relieve common symptoms
- Trials for which there is no ethically compelling need to monitor the interim comparisons of safety or efficacy

Further considerations that can impact a decision regarding the need for a DSMB or other monitoring entities include study size and study site. A study with a large sample size may best be monitored by a DSMB/DSMC/DMC, whereas a study with a small sample size may be monitored by an independent monitor (e.g., medical director or safety officer). Multicenter protocols may require a central DSMB/DSMC/DMC to monitor aggregate data while a single-site protocol may well use a local organization.

DSMBs/DSMCs/DMCs meet periodically, based on accrual targets or calendar intervals, to review every aspect of the study. Elements monitored may include but are not limited to

- The research protocol (e.g., study design), informed consent documents, and plans for data and safety monitoring
- Study progress (e.g., data quality and timeliness, subject recruitment, accrual and retention, changes in risk/benefit, and trial site performance)
- Relevant information regarding scientific and therapeutic developments with the actual or potential risk to impact study conduct and/or participant safety
- Data integrity
- Confidentiality of data
- Interim analysis of efficacy in accordance with stopping rules

The review, which may result in continuation, modification, or termination of a study, is documented in meeting minutes. The minutes should include the date of review and members present, a summary of adverse events with causality determinations, relevant literature reviews, and recommendations regarding study continuation, modification, suspension, or early stopping. Group reports are forwarded to the investigator(s) for review.

The PI is responsible for stating in the DSMP whether or not a DSMB/DSMC/DMC or additional monitoring entities will be in place for a particular protocol. Additionally, the investigator is responsible for providing information to the IRB about the qualifications/areas of expertise of group members, the nature and frequency of monitoring activities, interim analyses, and the preparation and distribution of reports. DSMB/DSMC/DMC reports are forwarded to the PI for submission to the IRB at the time of Continuing Review and more frequently, as indicated. A number of resources are available to provide additional information regarding the responsibilities and conduct of DSMB/DSMC/DMC (3–5).

The Role of the Institutional Review Board (IRB) in the Review and Approval of DSMPs?

The IRB has authority to approve, require modifications in, or disapprove all human research activities covered by federal regulations (see Chapter 2 for details). The committee of at least five members, with varying backgrounds, experience, and expertise, must determine at the time of initial and continuing review that all federal requirements for data and safety monitoring have been met. If requirements are met, the IRB has the authority to approve the study; if not met, the IRB has the authority to require modification of the protocol or to disapprove the research.

Included in both the IRB's initial and continuing reviews is the evaluation of the investigator's plan for data and safety monitoring. At the time of *initial review*, approval of the plan is contingent upon the adequacy of provisions for subject safety and data monitoring, the adequacy of the monitoring entity established, and the extent to which the provisions are commensurate with the nature, size, and complexity of the clinical trial. At the time of *continuing review*, the IRB evaluates all relevant information received from the PI and from monitoring entities since the date of its last review. The IRB makes a determination whether or not the data received alters its previous conclusion that the risks to subjects are minimized and are reasonable in relation to perceived benefits. Information submitted to the IRB by the investigator should address compliance with the DSMP and a summary of study progress (e.g., accruals, drop outs, withdrawals, patterns of adverse events and unanticipated problems, events occurring with greater frequency and/or severity than anticipated, patterns of protocol deviations and violations, interim findings, and changes in risk/benefit). Adverse events and the patterns of events are carefully reviewed to determine whether an adverse event has occurred in one or more subjects; is unexpected in nature, severity, or frequency; is related or possibly related to participation in the research suggesting that the research may be placing subjects or others at a greater physical or psychological harm than was previously known or recognized. In addition to onsite data, information and recommendations from other study sites and other monitoring entities should be submitted and evaluated, whether provided by a research sponsor, medical monitor, coordinating or statistical center, data and safety monitoring board, data safety monitoring committee, or data monitoring committee. Such information is invaluable to the IRB in making determinations regarding whether substantive changes in the research protocol or informed consent process/document or other corrective actions are warranted in order to protect the safety, welfare, or rights of research subjects (6).

CONCLUSIONS

It is the role and responsibility of the research investigator to protect human subjects. Not only is the researchers' number one ethical imperative, it is a federal mandate. The development of a comprehensive, integrated plan for monitoring study data and participant safety followed by rigorous compliance with and evaluation of the plan are critical. Such means safeguard human subjects, optimize the integrity, and meaning of study data and enhance the experience of participants in the research arena.

REFERENCES

1. Code of Federal Regulations. Available at: **http://www.hhs.gov/ohrp/humansubjects/guidance/45cfr46.htm**. Accessed May 26, 2010.
2. Code of Federal Regulations. Available at: **http://www.accessdata.fda.gov/scripts/cdrh/cfdocs/cfcfr/CFRSearch.cfm?CFRPart=56**. Accessed May 26, 2010.
3. NIH Policy for Data and Safety Monitoring. Available at: **http://grants.nih.gov/grants/guide/notice-files/not98-084.html**. Accessed May 26, 2010.
4. Guidance on Reporting Adverse Events to Institutional Review Boards for NIH-Supported Multicenter Trials. Available at: **http://grants.nih.gov/grants/guide/notice-files/not99-107.html**. Accessed May 26, 2010.
5. Further Guidance on Data and Safety Monitoring for Phase I and Phase II Trials. Available at: **http://grants.nih.gov/grants/guide/notice-files/NOT-OD-00-038.html**. Accessed May 26, 2010.
6. Office for Human Research Protections (OHRP)/Department of Health and Human Services (HHS)Guidance on Reviewing and Reporting Unanticipated Problems Involving Risks to Subjects or Others and Adverse Events. Available at: **http://www.hhs.gov/ohrp/policy/AdvEvntGuid.htm**. Accessed May 26, 2010.

CHAPTER 14

Presenting, Writing, and Publishing Challenges

Charles T. Quinn, MD, MS, and A. John Rush, MD

OUTLINE

INTRODUCTION

Articulate Writing Is Critical to Scientific Success

This chapter summarizes material presented in a course that we have taught at the University of Texas Southwestern Medical Center at Dallas. The material is a synthesis of material from a variety of sources (see References), to which we have added our own, sometimes idiosyncratic, suggestions for developing peer-reviewed journal reports of clinical and translational research. We particularly want to acknowledge *Essentials of Writing Biomedical Research Papers* by Mimi Zeiger (1) at the University of California at San Francisco, whose book we highly recommend.

    Writing clearly and accurately is critical to the success of your scientific career. If you do not write clearly, your article will not be cited. If you are not cited, you will not get promoted. If you do not get promoted, you will not have a job. Writing clearly to maximize your likelihood of being cited by others is key to your scientific survival. Published research is your only final product. A poorly written report could mean that you have wasted years conducting your study, because what you have done will not be cited or known. As such, it will not impact the field. The threat of career failure should be a powerful motivator for writing clearly, as is doing the very best science that one can.

Each article tells a story, but there is no "one true path" to writing. We each learn how to use our talents, overcome our deficiencies, and develop our skills differently. Each article we write is less difficult, but none is ever easy. To avoid feeling overwhelmed by the effort, we suggest that you approach writing as a series of questions to be clearly answered: What was the research question? Why does the answer matter? What was done? What was found? Has anyone else found that (or not)? What might it mean? What limitations or qualifications apply to the findings?

Define What to Report

What are you going to write? Obviously, the primary paper focuses on the main hypotheses that you tested. But there may be several secondary hypotheses and may be a couple of tertiary papers that are hypothesis generating. But be careful. Do not write trivial papers (third-rate papers with too small samples). They take too much time, are not cited, and have minimal to no payoff.

So, consider at the outset what aspects of the project are to be submitted, where, and in what order. What is the primary paper? Are there secondary papers? Clinical investigation often requires many people, so consider which colleagues might like to take the lead on a secondary paper. That is, depending on the size of the study and the contributions, needs, and expertise of your multidisciplinary research team, think about additional papers for others than yourself.

Getting Started

How often have you heard, "I have writer's block?" What does that mean? Everybody who has attended medical, dental, or nursing school can write. Thus, "writer's block" is a fiction—an excuse. The underlying fear may be that either one cannot think clearly enough to be able to say what was done (in which case, a career change is indicated!) or one is afraid that the product will not be "good enough" and therefore procrastinates.

To overcome "writer's block," simply realize at the outset that most of the words in the first draft will not make it to the final draft. Once you have something on paper, however, you can edit it—repeatedly. To get it on paper, dictate, type, or handwrite it (whatever is fastest for you). We recommend that you start with an outline. The outline is straightforward: title, abstract, introduction, methods, results (with tables and figures), discussion, conclusions, references, acknowledgments, and disclosures. Then write a topic sentence for each paragraph in each section. The outline and the topic sentences should take you about an hour-and-a-half to write. Then start to write each paragraph in the four key sections (introduction, methods, results, and discussion).

One place to begin is with the protocol that you followed to conduct the study. The protocol contains the aims, hypotheses/questions, rationale, and methods. Thus, the protocol

TABLE **14-1** | The Main Elements of a Manuscript

Elements	Length and Limits
Title	<12 words
Abstract	250–300 words
Introduction	600 words (3–4 paragraphs)
Methods	3–4 pages
Results	2–3 pages
Tables and figures	≤5 combined (see journal style)
Discussion	3–5 pages
References	<40 (see journal style)

is the basis for the first drafts of the introduction and methods. You may need to update the significance (to beef up the introduction) and to cite the newest relevant literature. Borrow from what you have done to begin.

Recall that most journals limit articles to 3000 to 4000 words. If each paragraph has 200 words, you have to write 18 to 20 paragraphs **(Table 14-1)**. The introduction has 3 to 4 paragraphs (never longer than 2 manuscript pages); discussion has 5; results typically has 4 to 6, depending on the number of questions; leaving 5 to 6 for methods. Once you break it down this way, it does not seem so bad.

Prepare to Spend Time

Realize that writing takes a lot of time. You must set aside uninterrupted time, which in our view is best inserted between other activities that do not involve writing. Write for a while, then stop and leave it alone. When you go back later, you will be more objective and be better able to edit your prior work. Too many people frustrate themselves by expecting to write up 4 years of work in 4 weeks. That is not realistic, especially if you have not written many prior papers, if you have other duties, or both. So think about what you want to produce and divide the work into "doable" pieces (e.g., the major sections noted above). Allocate a fixed amount of uninterrupted time each day to work on one section at a time to assemble these pieces without regard to how well it is written and without thinking about references. Simply tell the story.

Tell the Story

Look at the big picture first. Recall that you know more about what you have done than anybody else, so do not get nervous. You know the story—what you did and why you did it. Writing the first draft should not be a big thing. Polishing your drafts is where the time is.

The most important thing is to tell the story. Most people get stuck in the details and lose track of the story. Readers want to know what the issues were, why they matter, and what questions were asked (introduction). Then how were the issues addressed, questions answered, and hypotheses tested (methods)? Next, what were the answers (results)?

TABLE **14-2** | Elements of the Story Line

Element	Place in the Manuscript
Gaps in knowledge	Introduction
Hypotheses or questions addressed	Introduction, methods
What was done to test the hypotheses or answer the questions?	Methods
The answers to the questions	Results
The meaning of the answers	Conclusions

The results section is divided into subheadings, often based on the questions or hypotheses at the end of the introduction. A table or figure should accompany each question. Finally, what do you make of the results (discussion)? These are the major sections of each empirical report for scientific journals **(Tables 14-1** and **14-2).**

Recall for Whom You Are Writing

Do not write your paper for scientists, colleagues, the promotion and tenure committee, or your department chair. Tell the story as if you were talking to somebody who is not an expert in your area. If you make the article that simple and straightforward, readers will be able to understand what you did and be able to cite the paper. If you use a lot of jargon, compound sentences, or obscure wording, only you and your coauthors will actually know what you are saying.

Be Pithy

Table 14-3 highlights the most common reasons for rejection/revision. Most of these issues can be addressed by being pithy (succinct but full of substance and meaning) and consistent. Sentences should be simple: subject, verb, object, period. Whenever possible, avoid

TABLE **14-3** | Common Reasons for Rejection or Revision

Introduction too long
Methods lack detail
Results jumbled
Figures and tables not clear or not useful
Discussion too long
Confusing or inconsistent terminology
Manuscript too long (wordy)
Lack of flow
Does not "tell the whole story"

compound sentences. Do not change terminology throughout the paper (e.g., do not interchangeably use subjects, participants, patients, or volunteers). Readers will wonder why you changed the names. Whatever word or phrase you use to describe something, keep using the same term. This is not an English essay or creative-writing class. A scientific article uses an expository writing style—it simply tells the facts. The reader needs specificity, clarity, and brevity—not engaging phraseology. Be very specific. Avoid general statements such as, "The patients improved." What does that mean? Better to say something like "Patients in group A had a greater reduction in X than did patients in group B; test, P value (Table X)." Finally, physicians tend to be pompous in their style of writing. Avoid this; it prevents clear communication. Invest in a guide to clear medical writing to help (2).

Let us now consider each element in a manuscript.

THE MANUSCRIPT

Title

The title should have 12 words or fewer (pithy). Notice that movies do not have long titles. *The Fugitive*. Not *Escaping Jail Following an Unfair Conviction in Chicago*. Just *The Fugitive*.

Do not say: "A study of X." Of course it is a study. That wastes words. Begin the title with a key word. Be to the point. Grab the reader's attention. **Table 14-4** lists characteristics of a good title.

Abstract

There are two kinds of abstracts: structured and unstructured. Structured abstracts have distinct subsections: objectives, methods, results, and conclusions (these may vary by journal). Unstructured abstracts contain the same information, but are just one long paragraph.

Most people do not read an entire article. Everyone reads the abstract. So whatever is in the abstract is what everyone thinks is in the article. Therefore, it is critical to edit, polish, and perfect the abstract, because it is almost the only information that readers will take home.

What is the state of knowledge? What was the question (background)? What did you do and how did you do it (methods)? What did you find (results)? What is the bottom line (conclusion)? That's it!

TABLE **14-4** | Characteristics of a Good Title

Snappy, simple, short, concise, specific
Easy to understand
A headline (but an accurate promise)
Interesting, "a reader grabber"
Non declarative (do not give the conclusions)
Begin with a key word
Consider a question
No abbreviations (unless common to the journal)

TABLE **14-5** | **The Introduction: Start Broadly, Then Narrow**

Paragraph 1: What is known
Paragraph 2: What is unknown
Paragraph 3: What is the study question
Paragraph 4: What, briefly, is the experiment

We like to write the abstract first because it forces us to give the 10-second version of the paper. Then we polish it repeatedly after we write the article. The abstract will change a lot—often not substantively, but especially in terms of clarifying and simplifying the presentation. If you write your abstract first, you must ensure that it matches the final manuscript.

Introduction

At the beginning, tell the readers the problem **(Table 14-5)**. What do we know and what do we not know? Why does this matter? Then, what are the questions or hypotheses to be addressed or tested? What, in brief, was the approach?

The introduction should hook the reader. Paragraph no. 1: What is known? For example, "Diabetes is bad news, especially when it is associated with fatty liver." Paragraph no. 2: What is unknown? For example, "We do not know how to treat patients with this complication."

Paragraph no. 3: What is the question or hypothesis? "This study was conducted to determine whether A is better than B in improving fatty liver in patients with diabetes." What was done? "We addressed this question by conducting a randomized controlled trial of A versus B in diabetic patients with fatty liver." Be sure the introduction states your questions or hypotheses. End the introduction with a statement of your hypothesis: "We hypothesized that A was significantly better than B at decreasing fatty liver because. . . ." Bingo, the introduction is done.

The introduction is NOT a literature review. Do not over-reference. Seven to ten references are plenty. Less experienced writers seem to feel the need to cite the entire literature before getting to the methods. Do not. Everybody will trust that you can read. What they want to know is what was the issue. Why is it important? How did you approach the problem?

Methods

A poorly written methods section is a major reason for rejection. Be specific. Give details. Readers must know what you did. Remember, someone may try to replicate what you did! If the replication fails, your credibility is questioned. Give enough detail to ensure that another scientist can replicate exactly what you did. Give no more detail than is necessary, but give all the details that are required for replication.

The methods section is typically in chronological order. What did you do first? Then what did you do? Methods can be dense. Use subheadings in the text to guide the reader. **Table 14-6** lists common elements (subheadings) of methods.

T A B L E **14-6** | **Common Elements of the Methods**

Overview of study design
Participants (how gathered or recruited)
Eligibility (inclusion and exclusion)
Randomization and blinding
Interventions
Adherence and compliance measures
Concurrent treatments
Measurements
End points (outcomes)
Analyses

First, provide the study overview. What was the design? When was the study done? Where was it done? For example, "We conducted a multicenter randomized clinical trial of drug A versus placebo for 6 months in participants with type 2 diabetes and fatty liver." This brief, 30,000-ft overview primes the reader for the dense (but clear) text that follows.

Then provide the details **(Table 14-6)**. How did you recruit the sample? Consecutive? When you felt like it? How did you define who is eligible? When did the study start and stop? And so on. Do not include results in the methods section. The rules for obtaining the sample are in methods. The sample that you obtained by using these rules is described in the first paragraph of results (3,4). It is very important to say how the current sample relates to other reports of the same or related samples. Be very clear about whether patients in your study were or were not included in any prior reports. People doing meta-analyses or literature reviews, for example, must know whether the present sample is distinct or not from other samples. Surprisingly, you often cannot tell whether two reported samples are partially overlapping, the same, or distinct.

Describe where the study was conducted. Define all the variables used in the report, but none of the variables not in the report. Sometimes you might collect variables not included in this report. If they are in another report, you do not have to put them in this report.

What was the rationale for the randomization? Was it stratified? Was it computer based or did you use a table? Did you randomize in blocks? What was the informed consent process? Was there institutional review board or data safety monitoring board oversight? Were measurements blinded? Who was blinded and how?

How did you deliver the treatment of interest? How often were they treated? Who provided the treatment? How else were they managed? Could there be home visits? Could there be extra visits? Be very specific.

Did you assess whether patients adhered to treatment? If so, how? Did you ask them, count pills, or use MEMS caps?

How did you ensure that the people who delivered the study treatment did what they were supposed to do? Was there a manual? Was there quality control?

How were concomitant medicines managed? What rescue treatments or other efforts were used when patients worsened?

What were your outcomes or end points? Which was your primary outcome? Which were secondary? Who measured or obtained the end points? How? When? Was there quality control for these measures? Who did it? How? How often?

What sample size did you use? What kind of difference did you expect? What difference was expected? Did you power the study to detect this difference? What is the power? Why did you choose the statistical tests you did? Who did the analyses? Finally, it is very important that your coauthors see the data and have some discussion with the statistician so they really understand how the study was analyzed. You have to assume that your coauthors are going to make slides from this study and present it somewhere. If they do not understand the analysis, the audience will not. And they will be misinformed, unfairly judge your study, or both.

Results

When writing the results, we first build the tables and figures. Then we write the text to tell the story, answering the study questions, around the tables and figures. The text of results is often brief because the tables and figures provide the findings. Again, be pithy. The less you elaborate, the clearer you will be. You want the bottom line to be very, very clear. Remember, results is for the results. The introduction tells readers why you did the study. How you arrived at the results is in methods. What the results mean is in discussion.

Start with the results of the most important question, then the second most important, and so on. Or organize the section chronologically. Use subheadings to denote each question or section. There should be no interpretation of findings in results. Make the results exciting, but do not hype. **Table 14-7** lists important points to consider when writing this section.

If your patient sample is not extremely simple in composition, use a CONSORT chart (3,4). This chart explicitly and clearly shows how you obtained the evaluable sample. It will save you many words. Journals may require this chart, especially for clinical trials. If two (or more) groups were compared, describe and compare these groups at baseline. Serious adverse events, tolerability, attrition, and dosing may be in subsequent tables. Describe patients sensitively. People are not schizophrenics or diabetics. They are patients with schizophrenia or diabetes. They are participants, not subjects. Why participants? Because they chose to participate by giving consent. Subjects, such as rats, do not give consent (5).

TABLE **14-7** | The Results

Order results from the most to least important question
Order results chronologically (as they were performed
    in the experiments)
Key findings (from each study question) should be
    in tables and figures
Include final sample size and baseline characteristics
    (not in methods)

It is critical that the tables and figures carry the message. Do not repeat in the text what is in the tables and figures. Why? People can read the tables and figures. Use the text to direct the reader to the tables and figures. A sentence or two in the text to draw attention to a few key findings might be useful in the results section, but do not comment on every item in each table.

Tables and Figures

Figures and tables should stand alone. That is, each should be understood without reference to the text. The text simply alerts the reader when to look for them. So, if you use abbreviations or acronyms here, spell them out in the footnotes and legends. A figure has a title and legend that explains it; a table has a title and footnotes, if necessary, but no legend. Each figure or table should be on a separate sheet of paper. Remember, readers may use your tables and figures as slides. Make them clear and self-contained so that the slide has meaning.

Provide clear names for each column of your table. The study variables (e.g., age, sex, severe adverse events, and remission rates) are typically in the leftmost column, and each defines a row. The data are in the columns to the right. Avoid vertical lines in tables. The rows should have few to no horizontal lines.

Whenever you use a percentage in tables (and elsewhere), give the numerator and denominator so the reader can see how you derived it. We like to put significant P values in bold, but always follow journal style. Give the actual P value, not "NS" or "<0.05." Only use decimal places that are informative. For example, nobody knows what 48.134 years of age means. Report 48.1 years. Keep it simple.

Good figures are worth a thousand words and probably several tables. Figures should show your primary comparisons. The reader should be able to look at the figures and tables and know what the questions and answers are without reading the text. Avoid three-dimensional figures and gratuitous color and shading. Most of the ink used to print your table should represent your data, not explanatory or decorative material. Creating clear and meaningful figures is a skill one learns. Practice it. Texts by Tufte (6) and Goodman and Edwards (2) can aid you in good design.

Discussion

Next to the abstract, we find the discussion to be the most difficult part to write. We may be excited about what we have found and have lots to say about it. This may make the discussion wander. Here is a way to organize the discussion **(Table 14-8)**.

TABLE **14-8** | Elements of the Discussion

Synopsis of main results (order by study question)
Compare results to the literature and explain differences
Clinical and theoretical implications of findings (that is, so what?)
Limitations to study methods, certainty of results, and generalizability
Pithy conclusions

The first paragraph summarizes what you found. "This study was designed to determine whether A is better than B with regard to X. We found A was better than B in terms of tolerability, side effects, and remission rates, but not in terms of Y." If there was a second question, then the findings follow in the same first paragraph. You told them the questions (hypotheses) at the end of the introduction. Now, you summarize the answers. Avoid repeating the results; you just stated them.

The second paragraph of discussion addresses the question: "Has anybody else found anything like or different from what you found?" That is, how does it compare to the literature? If your findings are different, why? Is it the method, the sample, or measurement differences?

The third paragraph addresses the theoretical or clinical implications of the findings. What do these results mean about the utility or mechanisms of the study treatment or the pathophysiology of the disease being studied?

The fourth paragraph highlights limitations (and strengths). Limitations commonly include design, methods, generalizability, and internal validity. How certain are you about the results? A small study cannot be generalized. Measurements may have been too infrequent or too insensitive to detect an effect. Attrition may have been high. How does that affect certainty? Do not overstate the certainty of your findings. If you do not acknowledge the limitations of your report, the reviewers will make you. This is low-hanging fruit. Do not give reviewers the opportunity. Be honest, but this is your chance to frame the limitations in the best light. Remember, all studies have weaknesses. Do not feel embarrassed to list and discuss them. If your study has particular strengths, you may also highlight them here. This may soften the blow of the limitations.

Conclusions are pithy. Three sentences are enough—only one paragraph. A conclusion is "A is better than B for these kinds of patients. This conclusion is limited by X and Y." Some journals like you to suggest policy, economic, or practice implications—this is your final sentence: "Since X is better than Y and we have no other treatment for these patients, we recommend despite the limitations of this first trial that X might be a better treatment, but confirmatory studies are needed." A common phrase that ends the conclusion is "more studies are needed." Do not use it. More studies are always needed. Instead, state what studies you think are needed.

References

Leave the insertion of citations for the end. Where do references come up in the article? Largely in the introduction (7 to 10), methods (6 to 9), and discussion (15 to 20) (maximum, 30 to 40). The few references in the introduction should help lay out the problem and say why it is important. An introduction is NOT a literature review. The references in methods refer to measurements or techniques described in detail elsewhere. You do not have to describe them again; reference them.

If you use someone else's idea, give appropriate credit. Remember, that person could be a reviewer. You do not have to cite everything, just that which is immediately relevant to support your point. Rely on peer-reviewed literature, reports, and reviews.

Acknowledgments

Acknowledgments are undervalued by authors but highly valued by colleagues. Be generous. Cite those people who substantially assisted in the project (e.g., research assistants, key staff). Remember all the people who truly contributed to the success of the study, but who are not authors, and recognize them here.

Disclosures

Journals have different but increasingly strict rules about disclosure. Follow them closely. If you are in doubt about a relationship, disclose it. Only underdisclosing, not overdisclosing, will embarrass you.

GETTING IT PUBLISHED

Authorship

This is a thorny issue. If you are the principal investigator, we strongly advise that you meet with your study team when you launch a study to talk about authorship. Consider who will write up the primary question and key secondary questions. Talk it through early, so everybody knows the expectations from the beginning. This is especially important for junior faculty who need to know, after spending a couple of years on the study, what are they going to get out of it.

Who is supposed to be an author? Most journals have specific requirements. Those who have contributed to the design and execution of the project and helped in developing the manuscript are logical possible coauthors.

Just raising funds or being the chairman of the department does not qualify (use the acknowledgments for these individuals).

Typically, hired or support staff are not authors, but there may be exceptions, depending on their contributions. Students or fellows can certainly qualify if they make a substantive contribution either at the beginning, during the data analysis, or with the writing.

For large or multisite studies, it is extremely important to have a publication committee. Try to get on the publication committee. Some studies base authorship on enrollment, scientific expertise, execution of the study, and leadership. Have these discussions early and be up-front about authorship. Most people do not like to talk about authorship (as they do not like to talk about their salary). But you cannot be shy. Younger faculty need to be first, second, or third author. Beyond third author, you are "et al." Last is for senior authors.

RESEARCH ETHICS: PITFALLS & PRESCRIPTIONS

Even with the best of planning, authorship disputes can arise. For instance, senior mentors who permit a junior investigator use of lab or clinical space may feel entitled to coauthorship. The International Committee of Medical Journal Editors (www.icmje.org) offers excellent resources and guidelines for authorship status, editoral guidance, and related ethical issues in clinical research publishing. (In the above example, the ICMJE makes it clear that providing clinical/lab space does not justify coauthorship.)

TABLE **14-9** | Reasons to Rewrite

For organization and flow (the story)
For inclusion and exclusion of material
For clarity and necessity of tables and figures
For specificity and clarity of exposition
For wordiness, jargon, complex sentences, and phrases
For length
For references

Rewrites

Rewrites are critical. There are many reasons to rewrite **(Table 14-9)**. We suggest that you go after specific targets with each rewrite. If you have coauthors, use them. The first author should not have to write everything if coauthors are to merit the recognition. Once you get a draft, share it with coauthors and direct each one to a task. "X, please revise the introduction." "Y, please revise the methods." You distribute the work and have it come back to you. You have final editorial say as the first author. It also helps you to see how your coauthors interpret what you have written, what questions they have, and what changes they suggest.

When you ask coauthors to rewrite, set the time frame and tell them exactly what you want them to do. "Please give me feedback on the results section. Please review and revise within 7 days." Everybody has a large pile of things to do. Without a scheduled time limit, the article goes to the bottom of the pile. Rewrite one section at a time. Sequence the writers, so somebody does one section and someone else does another. But remember, the manuscript should not read as if there was a different author for each section. So, you have to ensure that the entire text "flows" and is stylistically consistent.

Table 14-9 shows areas of attention for rewrites. Shorten the introduction. Polish the abstract. Shorten the discussion. Double-check the methods to be sure the words are totally explicit, specific, and detailed. Delete jargon. Delete words. Make sure your tables and figures, if read alone, tell the results all by themselves.

Outside Readers

Once you and coauthors have written the article to its "final version," send it to two people who have no idea what you do, but who are intelligent and can communicate. They do not have to be experts in your area. Ask them to proofread the paper. Then ask them to tell you in their own words what you found. That way you will know whether they got the message.

Choosing a Journal

In choosing a journal, select one that is highly regarded with a high citation index. The journal content should match what you are reporting, so the readership will be interested in what you have to say. Some journals restrict length a lot—some less so, which might be a consideration in choosing a journal. Pick a journal as your first target that is bit of a long shot (sort of a stretch), but have in mind a second choice if the first rejects the paper. It is helpful if your second choice has similar requirements as the first. For example, you do not want to be limited to 4000 words for the first journal but to 2500 words for the second.

Rejections and Resubmissions

Rejections and negative reviews can be very frustrating. You may even feel angry or defeated. This is normal. Read the reviews through once, then put them aside for a while. If you are given the opportunity to resubmit, do not formulate your responses yet. Return several days later and read the reviews again. You will have a clearer mind then, and you will be less likely to respond angrily or with condescension. Some rejections are valid. Some are due to misunderstanding, which means that you were not clear. The reviewers took the time to read your article. If they did not "get it," it is your writing.

Sometimes the editorial response highlights the problem and seems to say either "Please fix this and resubmit" or "It's a long shot, but we'll re-review it if you want to try—no guarantee though." Always respond item-by-item to each of the reviewers' comments in a detailed letter. Be careful with your tone. A negative tone in your responses will work against you. We like to write the response letter before revising the paper. Think through everything you want to do, then revise the paper, and show your changes. Always include your coauthors in this process, because they are signing off on what you are resubmitting.

RESEARCH ETHICS: PITFALLS & PRESCRIPTIONS

The ethics of peer review is a complex topic. A peer reviewer, at minimum, should (a) show evidence of reading and comprehending the paper, (b) provide a rationale for objections or criticisms, and (c) hold the manuscript information and research data in confidence until the paper is published. Good peer reviewers summarize briefly the research aims, methods, and main conclusions of the paper; describe flaws of the project or manuscript clearly; and often sketch possible solutions to the identified problems. Authors receiving critical reviews often find themselves frustrated and angry, and this response should be tempered by the instructions in the main text. But in the situation where an author has a strong rationale for judging a review as unfair, this matter may be raised politely in the cover letter for the revised manuscript, pointing out the reasons why the author(s) believe the review was unfair. Most editors consider it impolitic for a revising author to make a specific request regarding an unfair review (such as throwing out the offending review, or requesting a new review) but all editors want fair-minded peer review for their journal, and authors' feedback in this arena can be helpful. Ultimately, the decision about a review and the fate of a manuscript is in the editor's hands, and the author's role is to make a persuasive case for the manuscript's acceptance.

CONCLUSION

We hope this synopsis is helpful. It took 15 drafts. It could still be better. So, writing is never easy. But what you want to get back from the reviewers is "This is a clearly written, succinct report of X. I have some remaining questions. . . ." No report is perfect. Recall that the reviewers are your helpers, but they cannot help improve your manuscript (or science) if you have not been clear in telling the story, specific in describing what you've done, and to the point throughout the paper. Good luck!

REFERENCES

1. Zeiger M. *Essentials of Writing Biomedical Research Papers*. 2nd ed. New York: McGraw-Hill; 1999.
2. Goodman NW, Edwards MB. *Medical Writing: A Prescription for Clarity*. 3rd ed. Cambridge, UK: Cambridge University Press; 2006.
3. Altman DG, Schulz KF, Moher D, et al. The revised CONSORT statement for reporting randomized trials: explanation and elaboration. *Ann Intern Med.* 2001;134:663–694.
4. Moher D, Schulz KF, Altman DG. The CONSORT statement: revised recommendations for improving the quality of reports of parallel-group randomized trials. *Ann Intern Med.* 2001;134:657–662.
5. Altman DG. Statistics and ethics in medical research: study design. *Br Med J.* 1980;281:1267–1269.
6. Tufte ER. *The Visual Display of Quantitative Information*. 2nd ed. Cheshire, CT: Graphics Press; 2001.

Informed Consent Template

In the document below, text denoting directions to the individual preparing the document are italicized.

Areas where text is to be added by the individual preparing the document are delineated by brackets.

CONSENT TO PARTICIPATE IN RESEARCH

Title of Research: [insert title]

Funding Agency / Sponsor: [name external funding source—if no external funds, state source of support]

Insert the names of the investigators and those individuals who will obtain consent

Study Doctors: [insert investigators names]

Research Personnel: [insert research personnel names]

You may call these study doctors or research personnel during regular office hours at [insert phone number]. At other times, you may call them at [insert after hours phone number].

Remove if not applicable.

Note: If you are a parent or guardian of a minor and have been asked to read and sign this form, the "you" in this document refers to the minor.

Instructions

Please read this consent form carefully and take your time making a decision about whether to participate. As the researchers discuss this consent form with you, please ask him/her to explain any words or information that you do not clearly understand. The purpose of the study, risks, inconveniences, discomforts, and other important information about the study are listed below. If you decide to participate, you will be given a copy of this form to keep.

Why is this study being done?

This study is being done to [please complete by adding brief rationale for conducting the proposed study]. *Sample language—'the study is being done to find out whether an investigational (non-FDA approved) drug called [insert drug name] can treat your condition better or more safely than standard medication'.*

Please note: If you are using an investigational drug, drug combination and/or device, please always indicate what is FDA approved and what is investigational, and define "investigational." For example: "The word 'investigational' means the [insert study drug or device or biologic] is still being tested in research studies and is not approved by the U.S. Food and Drug Administration (FDA)." Refrain from using "medicine," "treatment," or "therapy" for the investigational drug or device. Instead, use "study drug," "study procedures," "study processes," etc.

Why is this considered research?

This is a research study because [complete this sentence, assuring that all experimental or investigational drugs, devices, and/or procedures are clearly identified and defined].

Sample phrases for unapproved drugs, devices, or procedures:

- *[Insert drug/device name] is investigational and has not been approved by the U.S. Food and Drug Administration (FDA) for the treatment of [insert disease or condition].*
- *[Insert drug/device name] has been approved by the FDA to treat [insert approved use].*
- *[Insert drug name] is being compared to a standard drug, [insert standard drug name], that has already been approved by the FDA. The researchers are interested in learning which drug is more effective and/or safer in treating your condition/disorder.*
- *[Insert procedure] is being compared to the standard procedure [insert procedure here]. The researchers are interested in learning which procedure is more effective and/or safer in treating your condition/disorder.*

The following definitions may help you understand this study: *Delete definitions that do not apply to this study.*

- Double-blind means neither you nor the researchers will know which [insert applicable term: drug or device] you are receiving.
- Placebo controlled means that some participants will get a placebo. A placebo looks like the investigational drug but it includes no active ingredients (e.g., a sugar pill).
- Randomization means you will be placed by chance (like a flip of a coin) in one of the study groups. For studies with more than two arms, use "like drawing straws" instead of "flip of a coin."
- Single-blind means that you will not know which [insert applicable term: drug or device] you are receiving but the researchers will know.
- Standard medical care means the regular care you would receive from your personal doctor if you choose not to participate in this research.
- Researchers means the study doctor and research personnel at [insert names of institutions from which patients will be recruited] and its affiliated hospitals.

Why am I being asked to take part in this research study?

You are being asked to take part in this study because [outline briefly the reason this study is being conducted].

Sample Language:
You are being asked to take part in this study because you have high blood pressure.

Do I have to take part in this research study?

No. You have the right to choose whether you want to take part in this research study. If you decide to participate and later change your mind, you are free to stop participation at any time.

If you decide not to take part in this research study, it will not change your legal rights or the quality of health care that you receive at this center.

How many people will take part in this study?

About [insert number] people will take part in this study at [insert names of institutions from which patients will be recruited]. *If a multicenter trial, please also insert: "This study also is taking place at a number of other medical facilities around the country. There will be a total of [insert number] people participating in this research study throughout the United States and/or other countries."*

What is involved in the study?

If you volunteer to take part in this research study, you will be asked to sign this consent form and will have the following tests and procedures. Some of the procedures may be part of your standard medical care, but others are being done solely for the purpose of this study.

Screening procedures   To help decide if you qualify to be in this study, the researchers may ask you questions about your health, including medications you take and any surgical procedures you have had.

You may also have to fill out certain forms or have the following examinations, tests, or procedures:

Sample language

- *Physical examination and medical history;*
- *Vital signs;*
- *Blood tests;*
- *Electrocardiogram (EKG), a tracing of the electrical activity of the heart; and*
- *Demographic information (age, sex, ethnic origin).*

If applicable:

Group assignment   If the researchers believe you can take part in this study, you will be assigned randomly (like a flip of a coin) to receive either [insert study drug or procedure] or [insert placebo (inactive substance) or other study arm]. You have a [insert number] in [insert number] chance of receiving [insert name of the medication, device procedure, etc.] or placebo. *For studies with more than two arms, use "like drawing straws" instead of "flipping a coin."*

If applicable:

The group you will be in is decided by [insert who determines the randomization]. Neither you nor the researchers will be allowed to choose which group you are assigned to.

If the study is not blinded, please delete the following paragraph:

Neither you nor the researchers will know which group you are in. However, the sponsor will release the information about your assignment to the researchers if it is needed for your safety.

If applicable:

Study medication/intervention   [Insert description of the study medication or study intervention]

For example:

If you decide to participate in this study you will take either:

- *1 tablet of alpha-peg (10 mg) twice a day or*
- *1 tablet of pegatron (25 mg) twice a day.*

Procedures and evaluations during the research   *Explain the procedures and evaluations (as outlined in the protocol). Clearly identify any inconvenient, experimental, or painful procedures (such as long clinic visits, keeping a detailed diary between clinic visits, collection of multiple blood samples, etc.)*

Specify the amount of blood that will be drawn at any one time in teaspoons, tablespoons, or cups. Specify the number of study visits and the approximate length of time it will take to complete each study visit.

When describing what is involved in the study, please consider using a detailed timeline.

For example:

You will have the following tests and/or evaluations:

Visit 1:

- *Physical examination;*
- *An EKG; and*
- *Two tablespoons of blood will be drawn from your arm by needle stick for blood tests.*

Visit 2:

- *You will receive the study drug intravenously (into your vein) for 2 hours and*
- *You will complete two questionnaires.*

Or insert a simple table

The [insert research related test(s)] in this study are designed for research, not for medical purposes. They are not useful for finding problems or diseases. Even though the researchers are not looking at your [insert research related test(s)] to find or treat a medical problem, you will be told if they notice something unusual. You and your regular doctor can then decide together whether to follow up with more tests or treatment. Because the [insert research related test(s)] done in this study are not for medical purposes, the research results will not be sent to you or to your regular doctor.

Procedures for storing of extra or leftover samples   *Please note if DNA testing will be completed on the samples, a separate DNA Consent Form must be completed.*

Explain the procedures for the storing of the extra or leftover samples and the purpose of storing the samples. This information should include:

- *How the samples will be labeled;*
- *Whether or not identifiers will be kept;*
- *Location of where the samples will be kept; and*
- *Who will have access to the samples?*

Insert the following, if the study will collect and use the subject's social security number.

The researchers will record and use your Social Security Number (SSN) in order to [state intended use]. You do not have to give this information to the researchers; however, it may result in [state what may happen if the subject fails to provide SSN]. This information will remain confidential unless you give your permission to share it with others or if we are required by law to release it.

How long can I expect to be in this study?

Please describe here how long the study will be (in weeks, days, or months). Describe also (if applicable) whether you intend to collect follow-up information, and how much time that collection will require. For example, until 6 months after last study drug dose, for the rest of your life, etc.

You can choose to stop participating for any reason at any time. However, if you decide to stop participating in the study, we encourage you to tell the researchers. You may be asked if you are willing to complete some study termination tests.

What are the risks of the study?

Please note: The risk section should only contain the risks associated with study procedures. Risks of standard medical care procedures that are not required for this study should not be included in the consent form.

Please list only the risks and side effects related to the investigational aspects of the study and any standard of care procedures that are mandated for entry and during the course of the study. Any risks from standard medical care procedures that are not specially mandated should not be included.

For example: A patient who is undergoing joint replacement surgery for osteoarthritis, and the surgeon wants to participate in a trial of a new postoperative analgesic. The risks of the general anesthesia or orthopedic surgery do not need to be included in the Consent From. However, for a trial of a drug-eluting stents versus medical management, all of the risks regarding the stent procedure would need to be included even though the procedure is standard of care.

Study procedure/intervention   Because of your participation in this study, you are at risk of the following side effects. You should discuss these with the researchers and your regular health care provider.

[Insert study drug name] may cause some, all, or none of the side effects listed below.

Please list only the risks and side effects related to the investigational aspects of the study, and do not list side effects of supportive medications unless the medications are specifically mandated by the study.

Please insert a separate section for each study drug / device / procedure. Please include the frequency of the side effects in percentages. Large ranges, such as "2% to 60%" should be avoided. Since there is no standard definition of frequent, occasional, or rare, as a guide, "frequent" can be viewed as occurring in greater than 20% of subjects, "occasional" as 2% to 20% of subjects, and "rare" as less than 2% of subjects. However, frequencies may be adapted to specific study agents. If more specific data are not available, use the largest percent.
For example:

	Frequent (30% of subjects)	Occasional (15% of subjects)	Rare (less than 1% of subjects)
Serious		Blood clots in lungs	Death Irregular heart beat
Less serious	Low white blood cells	Moderate rash	Itching
Minor	Headache	Mild rash	
Trouble sleeping	Hiccups		

or

Frequent	Occasionally
• Headache	• Blood clots in lungs
• Trouble sleeping	• Moderate rash
Rare	Serious but rare
• Hiccups	• Death
	• Irregular heart beat

Psychological stress   *If the study involves psychological stress, please state.* Some of the questions we will ask you as part of this study may make you feel uncomfortable. You may refuse to answer any of the questions, take a break, or stop your participation in this study at any time.

Loss of confidentiality   Any time information is collected; there is a potential risk for loss of confidentiality. Every effort will be made to keep your information confidential; however, this cannot be guaranteed.

Please note: For class D medications please use the risk to an embryo or fetus language provided by the sponsor and the FDA instead of, or in addition to, the following template language in the "Risks to Sperm, Embryo, Fetus, or Breast-Fed Infant" section.

Risks to sperm, embryo, fetus, or breast-fed infant
Males: Being in this research may damage your sperm, which could cause harm to a child that you may father while on this study. If you take part in this study and are sexually active, you must agree to use a medically acceptable form of birth control. Medically acceptable forms of birth control include:

(1) Surgical sterilization (vasectomy) or
(2) A condom used with a spermicide (a substance that kills sperm).

Females: If you are part of this study while pregnant or breast-feeding an infant, it is possible that you may expose the unborn child or infant to risks. For that reason, pregnant and breast-feeding females cannot participate in the study. If you can become pregnant, a blood pregnancy test will be done (using 1 teaspoon of blood drawn from a vein by needle stick), and it must be negative before you participate in this study. If you take part in this study and you are sexually active, you and any person that you have sex with must use medically acceptable birth control (contraceptives) during the study. Medically acceptable birth control (contraceptives) includes:

(1) Surgical sterilization (such as hysterectomy or "tubes tied"),
(2) Approved hormonal contraceptives (such as birth control pills, patch or ring; Depo-Provera, Depo-Lupron, Implanon),
(3) Barrier methods (such as condom or diaphragm) used with a spermicide (a substance that kills sperm), or
(4) An intrauterine device (IUD).

If you do become pregnant during this study, you must tell the researchers immediately.
If the study will include exposure to radiation, please include the following:
Radiation exposure to a woman's reproductive organs may harm an embryo or fetus. Also, if radioactive materials are used for certain types of scans, harm may come to an embryo, fetus, or an infant who is breast-feeding.

Pregnancy tests performed during the early stages of pregnancy do not always reveal pregnancy. Therefore, radiation exposure that includes the reproductive organs will be limited to the first 10 days after a woman who can become pregnant (age 10 to 50 years) has begun her most recent menstrual period. This is a standard policy in clinics and hospitals within [insert names of institutions from which patients will be recruited]. This policy applies unless there is an important medical reason requiring radiation outside this time frame.

If minors will be enrolled in the study, please insert the following:
If your parents or guardian asks, we will tell them the results of your pregnancy test or that you are using birth control.

Risks of radiation—diagnostic test   *Insert the risk statement if applicable to your study.*

If the amount of radiation exposure is the same regardless as to whether the participant elects to participate in this research study or receives standard medical care, please include the following sentence. The radiation dose that you will get from diagnostic tests is medically indicated for your condition, and it is the same that you would get if you were not involved in this research study.

If the amount of radiation exposure is more than the participant would receive if they elected to receive standard medical care, please include one of the following sentences.

If additional radiation dose < 350 mrem from research:
This research study includes exposure to radiation from diagnostic tests in addition to that you would receive from standard care. The additional radiation dose you will get is about [insert percentage from table] % of the average radiation dose from all sources (natural background radiation, consumer appliances, radon gas, medical tests, etc.) that a person in the United States receives each year. (The exact wording and estimate should be defined by consultation with local [institutional] Radiation Safety Committee or equivalent administrative office.)

If additional radiation dose > 350 mrem from research:

This research study includes exposure to radiation from diagnostic tests in addition to that you would receive from standard care. The risk of harm to your body from this radiation can be compared to risks from everyday activities. For example, the risk of developing fatal cancer during your lifetime from this radiation is comparative to the risk of suffering a fatal car crash while driving [XX] miles in an automobile. The average household in the United States drives 23,000 miles per year (2001 data). (The exact wording and estimate should be defined by consultation with local [institutional] Radiation Safety Committee or equivalent administrative office.)

If additional radiation dose involving cardiac catheterization, electrophysiology studies, interventional peripheral and neuroradiology procedures, the investigator should consult with a medical physicist to determine if additional statements covering any deterministic effects—such as erythema or epilation—may be required.

Risks of radiation—radiation therapy   *If the amount of radiation exposure is the same regardless as to whether the participant elects to participate in this research study or receives standard medical care, please include the following text.*

The radiation therapy used in this research is the standard radiation therapy for your health problem; therefore, the risk of harm to your body is the same. Your radiation doctor will discuss the known risks of radiation therapy with you and ask you to sign a separate specific treatment site consent form.

High-dose radiation treatments to or near a man's testicles or a woman's ovaries may produce harmful changes that could be passed on to children through a sperm or an egg.

Women: Females (ages 10 to 50 years) able to have children should avoid becoming pregnant until after they have had three menstrual periods after the end of all radiation therapy. After three menstrual periods, there is almost no risk of harmful changes to an egg.

Men: Males must avoid fathering a child until 10 weeks after the end of all radiation therapy. After that period, there is much less risk of harmful changes to sperm. Even then there is still an unknown amount of risk.

Possible side effects of radiation therapy to the (site) include: (select the appropriate short- and long-term effects from risk information that will be available by consultation with the local [institutional] Radiation Safety Committee. The exact wording and estimate should be defined by consultation with this committee).

If the amount of radiation exposure is different from the standard of care, please include the following sentence.

The radiation therapy in this research is different from the standard radiation therapy for your health problem. The radiation dose that will be used is (more/less/given in a different way) than the standard treatment. The potential risks of this dose include: [consult with radiation oncologist for assistance].

Risks of blood drawing   *Insert the risk statement if applicable to your study*

Risks associated with drawing blood from your arm include minimal discomfort and/or bruising. Infection, excess bleeding, clotting, and/or fainting also are possible, although unlikely.

If blood samples are collected as part of the participants' standard medical care, please include the following sentence. You will have the same amount of blood collected whether you receive standard medical care for your health problem or take part in this research.

If blood samples are collected solely for the purpose of research, please include the following sentence. You will have [insert amount in lay terms] of blood collected because you are in this research study.

If applicable:

Placebo   If you receive a placebo, you will not receive active medication for your health problem. If your problem becomes worse, your participation in the research will stop. If this happens, your study doctor can discuss alternative care with you.

Note: The amount of blood that can be collected may differ from institution to institution and is defined locally by individual IRBs. In adults, this is a relatively large volume and may be modified by the presence of anemia or other intercurrent illnesses. In the pediatric age groups, this quantity is more restricted and varies by age and weight. These volumes and frequencies should be obtained from the local institutional IRB office.

Other Risks   There may possibly be other side effects that are unknown at this time. If you are concerned about other, unknown side effects, please discuss this with the researchers.

How will risks be minimized or prevented?

Describe how the study design and procedures will prevent and / or minimize any potential risks or discomfort. Potential risks and discomforts must be minimized to the greatest extent possible by using procedures such as appropriate training of personnel, monitoring, or withdrawal of the subject upon evidence of difficulty or adverse event and referral for treatment, counseling, or other necessary follow-up.

What will my responsibilities be during the study?

While you are part of this study, the researchers will follow you closely to determine whether there are problems that need medical care. It is your responsibility to do the following:

- Ask questions about anything you do not understand.
- Keep your appointments.
- Follow the researchers' instructions.
- Let the researchers know if your telephone number or address changes.
- Store study materials [insert tablets, vials of liquid, needles, etc. as applicable] in a secure place at home away from anyone who is unable to read and understand labels, especially children.
- Tell the researchers before you take any new medication, even if it is prescribed by another doctor for a different medical problem or something purchased over the counter.
- Tell your regular doctor about your participation in this study.
- If study involves medication, please state. Carry information about [the research medication] in your purse or wallet.
- Report to the researchers any injury or illness while you are on study even if you do not think it is related.

If I agree to take part in this research study, will I be told of any new risks that may be found during the course of the study?

Yes. You will be told if any new information becomes available during the study that could cause you to change your mind about continuing to participate or that is important to your health or safety.

What should I do if I think I am having problems?

If you have unusual symptoms, pain, or any other problems while you are in the study, you should report them to the researchers right away. Telephone numbers where they can be reached are listed on the first page of this consent form.

If you have a sudden, serious problem, like difficulty breathing or severe pain, go to the nearest hospital emergency room, or call 911 (or the correct emergency telephone number in your area). Tell emergency personnel about any medications you are taking, including any medications you are taking for this study.

What are the possible benefits of this study?

Please note: The description of benefits to the participant should be clear and not overstated. If no direct benefit is anticipated, then that should be stated. If these benefits may be materially relevant to a participant's decision to participate, the benefits should be disclosed in the informed consent document.

If you agree to take part in this study, there [may or may not] be direct benefits to you. The researchers cannot guarantee that you will benefit from participation in this research.

We hope the information learned from this study will benefit others with [insert condition] in the future. Information gained from this research could lead to better [insert appropriate term, such as 'care', 'prevention', or 'treatment'].

What options are available if I decide not to take part in this research study?

If a treatment study, insert: You do not have to participate in this research to receive care for your medical problem. Instead of being in this study, you have the following options:

- [Please insert all alternative treatment options available to the participant] *Please note: When applicable, this should include receiving the study drug or treatment off study or the possibility of no treatment at all.*

Please talk to the researchers or your personal doctor about these options.

If not a treatment study, insert: This is not a treatment study. You do not have to be part of it to get treatment for your condition.

Will I be paid if I take part in this research study?

Yes. *Please explain what the participant will receive.*

Sample language 1:

You will be paid $100.00 at the end of the study. If you stop taking part in this study or are withdrawn by the research team, you will receive payment for only the visits you have completed. For example, if you complete four study visits you will be paid $40.00.

Sample language 2:

You will be given a $50.00 gift card to Toys R US at the end of the study if you take part in this research.

Sample language 3:

> *You will be given the following, if you take part in this research:*

- *XYZ tote bag;*
- *XYZ T-shirt; and*
- *XYZ notepads.*

If applicable:

There are no funds available to pay for parking expenses, transportation to and from the research center, lost time away from work and other activities, lost wages, or child care expenses.

Insert the following, if participant will receive a cash payment, their social security number will be collected.

Your Social Security Number (SSN) will be given to [insert name of host institution] in order to process your payment as required by law. This information will remain confidential unless you give your permission to share it with others, or if we are required by law to release it.

Insert the following, if participant will receive a cash payment.

If you are an employee of [insert name of host institution], your payment will be added to your regular paycheck and income tax will be deducted.

If applicable:

[insert name of host institution], as a State agency, will not be able to make any payments to you for your participation in this research if the State Comptroller has issued a "hold" on all State payments to you. Such a "hold" could result from your failure to make child support payments or pay student loans, etc. If this happens, [insert name of host institution] will be able to pay you for your taking part in this research (1) after you have made the outstanding payments and (2) the State Comptroller has issued a release of the "hold."

Insert the following, if participants will receive reimbursement for travel expenses, parking, etc.

You will be reimbursed for your parking expenses, transportation to and from the research center (e.g., cab or bus fare), or child care expenses. In order to receive reimbursement, you will need to turn in all your receipts to the research coordinator.

If participants will not be compensated, please delete the above paragraphs and insert: No. You will not be paid to take part in this research study. There are no funds available to pay for parking expenses, transportation to and from the research center, lost time away from work and other activities, lost wages, or child care expenses.

Will my insurance provider or I be charged for the costs of any part of this research study?

No. Neither you nor your insurance provider will be charged for anything done only for this research study (i.e., the Screening Procedures, Experimental Procedures, or Monitoring/Follow-up Procedures described above).

However, the standard medical care for your condition (care you would have received whether or not you were in this study) is your responsibility (or the responsibility of your insurance provider or governmental program). You will be charged, in the standard manner, for any procedures performed for your standard medical care.

Please note: If the participant's insurance company will be responsible for any research-related costs, please use the following language.

Yes. The costs of [insert items] will be billed to you or your insurance provider. We expect the costs of [insert items] to be [insert amount].

What will happen if I am harmed as a result of taking part in this study?

It is important that you report any illness or injury to the research team listed at the top of this form immediately.

Compensation for an injury resulting from your participation in this research is not available from [insert name of host institution] or [insert other institutions, if applicable].

If applicable: The sponsor has expressed a willingness to help pay the medical expenses necessary to treat such injury.

You retain your legal rights during your participation in this research.

Can I stop taking part in this research study?

Yes. If you decide to participate and later change your mind, you are free to stop taking part in the research study at any time.

If you decide to stop taking part in this research study, it will not affect your relationship with the [insert name of host institution] staff or doctors. Whether you participate or not will have no effect on your legal rights or the quality of your health care.

If you are a medical student, fellow, faculty, or staff at [insert name of host institution], your status will not be affected in any way.

Include if recruiting from investigator's own patients:

Your doctor is a research investigator in this study. S/he is interested in both your medical care and the conduct of this research study. At any time, you may discuss your care with another doctor who is not part of this research study. You do not have to take part in any research study offered by your doctor.

If I agree to take part in this research study, can I be removed from the study without my consent?

Yes. The researchers may decide to take you off this study if:

- Your medical problem remains unchanged or becomes worse.
- The researchers believe that participation in the research is no longer safe for you.
- The researchers believe that other treatment may be more helpful.
- The sponsor or the FDA stops the research for the safety of the participants.
- The sponsor cancels the research.
- You are unable to keep appointments or to follow the researcher's instructions.

Will my information be kept confidential?

Insert this section for studies without a Certificate of Confidentiality.

Information about you that is collected for this research study will remain confidential unless you give your permission to share it with others, or if we are required by law to release it. You should know that certain organizations that may look at and/or copy your medical records for research, quality assurance, and data analysis include:

- [Insert sponsor's name];
- Representatives of government agencies, like the U.S. Food and Drug Administration (FDA), involved in keeping research safe for people; and
- The [insert name of host institution] Institutional Review Board.

In addition to this consent form, you will be asked to sign an "Authorization for Use and Disclosure of Protected Health Information." This authorization will give more details about how your information will be used for this research study, and who may see and/or get copies of your information.

Insert this section for studies with a Certificate of Confidentiality:
Information about you that is collected for this research study will remain confidential unless you give your permission to share it with others, or as described below. You should know that certain organizations that may look at and/or copy your medical records for research, quality assurance, and data analysis include:

- [Insert sponsor's name];
- Representatives of government agencies, like the U.S. Food and Drug Administration (FDA), involved in keeping research safe for people; and
- The [insert name of host institution] Institutional Review Board.

In addition to this consent form, you will be asked to sign an "Authorization for Use and Disclosure of Protected Health Information." This authorization will give more details about how your information will be used for this research study, and who may see and/or get copies of your information.

To help us further protect the information, the investigators will obtain a Certificate of Confidentiality from the U.S. Department of Health and Human Services (DHHS). This Certificate adds special protections for research information that identifies you and will help researchers protect your privacy.

With this Certificate of Confidentiality, the researchers cannot be forced to disclose information that may identify you in any judicial, administrative, legislative, or other proceeding, whether at the federal, state, or local level. There are situations, however, where we will voluntarily disclose information consistent with state or other laws, such as:

- To DHHS for audit or program evaluation purposes;
- Information regarding test results for certain communicable diseases to the Texas Department of State Health Services, including, but not limited to HIV, Hepatitis, Anthrax, and Smallpox;
- If you pose imminent physical harm to yourself or others;
- If you pose immediate mental or emotional injury to yourself;
- If the researchers learn that a child has been, or may be, abused or neglected; or
- If the researchers learn that an elderly or disabled person has been, or is being, abused, neglected, or exploited.

The researchers will not, in any case, disclose information about you or your participation in this study unless it is included in the Authorization for Use and Disclosure of Protected Health Information for Research Purposes as stated above.

The Certificate of Confidentiality does not prevent you or a member of your family from voluntarily releasing information about your involvement in this research study. In addition, the researchers may not use the Certificate to withhold information about your participation in this research study if you have provided written consent to anyone allowing the researchers to release such information (including your employer or an insurance company). This means that you or your family must also actively protect your privacy.

A Certificate of Confidentiality does not represent an endorsement of this research project by the Department of Health & Human Services or any other Federal government agency.

Are there procedures I should follow after stopping participation in this research?

Include this section if there are procedures to be followed or risks to participants after stopping participation in the research study.

Please specify what a participant will be asked to do in the event of early withdrawal from the study. Identify any materials (study pills, injections, liquids, creams, etc.) that need to be returned.

If applicable, please explain that sudden discontinuation of the study medication (such as corticosteroids or antipsychotic medications) or study device could be unsafe.

For example:

Yes. If you, the researchers, or the sponsor stops your participation in the research, you may be asked to do the following:

- *Let the researchers know immediately that you wish to withdraw from the research.*
- *Return to the research center for tests that may be needed for your safety.*
- *Return any unused study materials, including empty containers.*
- *Discuss your future medical care, if any, with the researchers and/or your personal doctor.*

If applicable, please include:

Is there anything else I should know before I decide?

[Insert name(s)] has/have financial interests in the company sponsoring this study. You should feel free to ask questions about this.

Whom do I call if I have questions or problems?

For questions about the study, contact [insert PI's name here] at [insert PI's number here with area code] during regular business hours and at [insert PI's 24-hour number here with area code] after hours and on weekends and holidays.

For questions about your rights as a research participant, contact the [insert name of host institution] Institutional Review Board (IRB) Office at xxx-xxx-xxxx.

SIGNATURES

YOU WILL BE GIVEN A COPY OF THIS CONSENT FORM TO KEEP

Your signature below certifies the following:

- You have read (or been read) the information provided above.
- You have received answers to all of your questions and have been told who to call if you have any more questions.
- You have freely decided to participate in this research.
- You understand that you are not giving up any of your legal rights.

_____

Participant's Name (printed)

_____   _____

Participant's Signature   Date

_____

Legally Authorized Representative's Name (printed)

_____   _____

Legally Authorized Representative's Signature   Date

_____

Name of person obtaining consent (printed)

_____   _____

Signature of person obtaining consent   Date

If applicable:
ASSENT OF A MINOR:

I have discussed this research study with my parent or legal guardian and the researchers, and I agree to participate.

_____   _____

Signature of participant (age 10 through 17)   Date

If applicable:
INTERPRETER STATEMENT:

I have interpreted this consent form into a language understandable to the participant, and the participant has agreed to participate as indicated by their signature on the associated short form.

_____   _____

Name of Interpreter (printed)

_____   _____

Signature of Interpreter   Date

Documentation
of Informed Consent

Initial Informed Consent and/or Revisions to Informed Consent: Study _____ _____	Was the subject **able to understand** and **willing** to give informed consent?	Did the subject **sign the ICF prior** to any **screening** activities or **implementation of protocol revisions?**	The **ICF version date** and **date signed by subject** and/or their **representative**
Initial Informed Consent ____English ____Spanish	____YES ____NO, specify	____YES ____NO, specify	ICF version _____/_____/_____ Date Signed _____/_____/_____ Copy given to Patient _____
Revised Informed Consent/Addenda ____English ____Spanish	____YES ____NO, specify	____YES ____NO, specify	ICF version _____/_____/_____ Date Signed _____/_____/_____ Copy given to Patient _____
Supplemental Information Provided to Patient– **Date** _____	_____ Written	____Verbal	Comment:

Signed _____   Date _____

Checklist for Assessing the Informed Consent Form

Does the Informed Consent Form contain the following required element?

(if No, add needed content on line below)

Yes **No**

❏ ❏ The name/nature and purpose of a proposed treatment or procedure

❏ ❏ The benefits of proposed treatment or procedures

❏ ❏ The risks of proposed treatment or procedures

❏ ❏ Alternatives (regardless of costs or extent covered by insurance)

❏ ❏ The risks and benefits of alternatives

❏ ❏ The risks and benefits of not receiving treatments or undergoing procedures

Does the form contain details (or space) for the following content?

Yes **No**

❏ ❏ Name and signature of the patient, or if appropriate, legal guardian;

❏ ❏ Name of the hospital;

❏ ❏ Name of all practitioners performing the procedure and individual significant task if more than one practitioner;

❏ ❏ Date and time consent is obtained;

❏ ❏ Statement that procedure was explained to patient or guardian;

❏ ❏ Space to document that patient is unable to speak English;

❏ ❏ Space for documentation of interpretive services (on site, telephonic, video) and/or of sight translation of form;

❏ ❏ Signature of professional person witnessing the consent; and

❏ ❏ Name and signature of person who explained the procedure to the patient

Other comments, questions, or suggestions you have about this Form:

_____

_____

_____

_____

_____

_____

_____

_____

_____

Genetic Informed Consent Template

In the document below, text denoting directions to the individual preparing the document are italicized.

Areas where text is to be added by the individual preparing the document are delineated by brackets.

[Institutions where research is to be conducted]

CONSENT TO PARTICIPATE IN RESEARCH

Title of Research: [insert title]

Funding Agency/Sponsor: [name external funding source—if no external funds, state source of support]

Please insert the names of the investigators and those individuals who will obtain consent.

Study Doctors: [insert investigators names]

Research Personnel: [insert research personnel names]

You may call these study doctors or research personnel during regular office hours at [insert phone number]. At other times, you may call them at [insert after hours phone number].

Remove if not applicable.

Note: If you are a parent or guardian of a participant younger than 18 years of age and have been asked to read and sign this form, the "you" in this document refers to the participant.

Instructions   Please read this consent form carefully, and take your time making a decision about whether to participate. As the researchers discuss this consent form with you, please ask him/her to explain any words or information that you do not clearly understand. The purpose of the study, risks, inconveniences, discomforts, and other important information about the study are listed below. If you decide to participate, you will be given a copy of this form to keep.

What is DNA?   DNA means *deoxyribonucleic acid*. DNA is the substance in our cells, which contains information we inherited from our parents and other family members. Your DNA contains "genes" that predict things like physical characteristics (eye color, hair color, height, etc.) and may also be a factor in whether you develop or are at risk of developing certain illnesses or disorders.

203

What is genetic testing?   Genetic tests look for naturally occurring differences in a person's genes, or the effects of specific genes. These differences could indicate an increased chance of getting a disease or condition. Genetic testing includes gene tests (DNA testing) and sometimes biochemical tests (protein testing) if it relates to a specific gene.

In gene tests, DNA in cells taken from a person's blood, body fluids, or tissues is examined for differences. The differences can be relatively large—a piece of a chromosome, or even an entire chromosome, missing or added. Sometimes the change is very small—as little as one extra, missing, or altered chemical within the DNA strand. Genes can be amplified (too many copies), overexpressed (too active), inactivated, or lost altogether. Sometimes pieces of chromosomes become switched, turned over, or discovered in an incorrect location.

Why is this study being done?   This study is being done to [please complete by inserting a description of the rationale for the study].
Sample phrases:

- *Find out more about [insert medical problem]. This research is being done because [insert rationale].*
- *Collect information about [insert medical problem] that will be used to better understand how genes may cause diseases and help doctors in their diagnosis and treatment.*
- *Create and maintain a tissue databank, which will use tissue, and cell and fluid samples for medical research designed to improve the understanding and treatment of [insert medical problem(s)].*

Why am I being asked to take part in this research study?   You are being asked to take part in this study because [insert reason/condition or eligibility criterion].
Sample language:
You are being asked to take part in this study because you or your relative has a problem with [insert medical problem].

You are being asked to take part in this tissue database because you or your relative has a problem with [insert medical problem].

How many people will take part in this study?   About [insert number] people will take part in this study at [insert names of institutions from which patients will be recruited]. *If a multicenter trial, please also insert:* This study is also taking place at a number of other medical facilities around the country. There will be a total of [insert number] people participating in this research study throughout the United States and/or other countries.

What is involved in the study?   If you agree to be in this study, you will be asked to sign this consent form and will have the following test and procedures.
If the study is a tissue repository and will be utilizing medical waste, the above paragraph can be deleted and the following paragraph may be inserted.

You will be undergoing a [insert procedure] procedure for [insert medical problem] that your doctor has discussed with you. This procedure has been deemed medically necessary, and you have agreed to the procedure. During that procedure certain tissues that are important to our studies will be obtained by your doctor. These tissues (i.e., operative specimens, blood, and bodily fluids) are often removed at the time of the pro-cedure, and extra pieces of tissue will be obtained for research purposes. Participation in this research will mostly involve using what is called "medical waste." Medical waste is leftover tissue and fluid that are not needed for diagnosis, and otherwise would be discarded.

Please revise the section below to clearly outline the information and samples being collected:

- **Questions:** [Insert name of investigator] will ask you questions about [describe types of questions that will be asked].
- **Samples of blood:** Up to [insert number] teaspoons of blood will be drawn from a vein in your arm with a small sterile needle. This is the standard method used to obtain blood for routine hospital tests. We may ask for a second blood sample if the research laboratory cannot process the first sample. *Sample language if the study is a tissue databank.* We would like to keep any leftover blood sample that would other-wise be discarded. If a sample does not exist, we would like to obtain an additional blood sample. The amount collected will be [insert number] teaspoons or less.
- **Samples of bodily fluids:** We would also like to obtain a sample of your [insert sample type]. We will collect [insert a description of what is being collected and the amount.] *Sample language if the study is a tissue databank.* We would like to keep any leftover [insert sample type] that would otherwise be discarded.
- **Samples of tissue.** We would like to obtain a sample of your [insert sample type]. We will collect [insert a description of what is being collected and the amount]. This extra sample is being collected only for research purposes and is not as part of your standard of care.
- **Cells removed during surgery:** If you have surgery for [insert medical condi-tion], we will keep some of the cells already removed during the surgery for research. If a sample already exists, which can be used in the study, we will attempt to use it.
- **Skin tissue biopsy:** We would like to obtain a small piece of skin (less than 1/8″) to be used for DNA analysis, culture of skin cells, microscopic study of the skin, or other laboratory tests. The skin will be removed using a local anesthetic (numbing medication) and a special instrument called a "punch."
- **Medical record:** You are also being asked for permission to obtain from your medical records information about your history and treatment that will make your tissue samples even more useful to the research community.

Please delete the following unless the study is a tissue repository.

By agreeing to participate in this research, you agree to be included in this research database. Investigators may use your health information for future research on various diseases including genetic research. However, your personally identifiable information will never be released to researchers, so they will not know who you are or be able to con-tact you.

Insert the following, if the study will collect and use the subject's social security number.

The researchers will record and use your Social Security Number (SSN) in order to [state intended use]. You do not have to give this information to the researchers; however, it may result in [state what may happen if the subject fails to provide SSN]. This information will remain confidential unless you give your permission to share it with others, or if we are required by law to release it.

How will my samples be identified?   Please describe how the samples will be identified:

This information should include:

- *How the samples will be labeled;*
- *Whether or not identifiers will be kept;*
- *Location of where the samples will be kept; and*
- *Who will have access to the samples?*

Insert if applicable: To protect your information, personally identifiable information will be kept in a secure facility with limited access and password protection. The computer maintained by [insert host institution name] is protected by a firewall that prevents unauthorized access to the information. Any results collected will not be released in a personally identifiable manner, and thus no information will be given to your insurance provider, employer, family, etc. without your permission.

Insert if applicable: Your sample will be marked with a coded identifier and will not be personally identifiable. Neither your name nor any identifying information will be given to the researchers who receive your samples.

How long can I expect to be in this study?   In many genetic studies, testing of the DNA

may go on for very long periods of time. This is true because we are continually finding new genes that may be involved in [insert medical problem]. Therefore, while your direct participation in this study will be over once you have completed the procedures/visits described above; the DNA isolated from your blood/tissue sample may continue to be studied for many years.

Can I stop taking part in this research study?   Yes. If you decide to participate and later

change your mind, you are free to stop taking part in the research study at any time. You may ask [insert name of investigator] to destroy any record of your participation in this research and to destroy any sample with your name on it. You will not be asked for further information or samples. Your identity will be removed from all research records. However, the resulting data from the research will not be discarded. Deidentified copies of DNA and/or growing cells made from your samples will not be destroyed.

Delete if not applicable. Samples sent to other scientists cannot be identified and destroyed because your name was removed before the samples were shipped to other medical centers.

What will happen to the samples collected for this research?

[Insert name of investigator] will compare information about the health of participants with the results of research tests using their DNA.

Delete if not applicable. Your blood/tissue sample will be used to isolate DNA for genetic analysis. Part of your blood/tissue sample will also be used to grow a long-term cell line. This immortalized cell line, called a lymphoblastoid cell line (or fibroblast cell line), will be stored in a Cell Bank and will be available for research, both now and in the future. This also allows us to perform many tests without having to ask you for additional blood/tissue samples.

How is DNA obtained?

Cells from blood or other body materials are processed in a laboratory that has special equipment that can extract DNA and identify genes.

How long will my samples be kept?

[Insert name of investigator] will keep your sample in a research laboratory at this medical center until it is all gone, becomes unusable, or until [insert he, she, or they] decides to discard the sample.

If your sample remains stored beyond your lifetime, your sample will be used as described in this document.

May other researchers use my sample?

When you provide a sample for purposes of this study your sample becomes the property of [Insert institution name] and may be used for future studies or provided to other investigators at other medical research facilities without any identifiers.

Who decides which research scientists may receive samples of my DNA?   [Insert name of investigator or group] will decide which researchers at this medical center and at other medical centers may receive samples of your DNA. Your samples may be used in other research only if the other research has been reviewed and approved by an Institutional Review Board (IRB).

Could my sample be used for other purposes?

No. Your samples or your DNA will only be used for research.

Research tests using your sample may possibly result in inventions or procedures that have commercial value and are eligible for protection by a patent.

Compensation for any future commercial developments is not available from the [Insert Institution name], its researchers or other facilities, or researchers whose research may benefit from the use of your sample.

By agreeing to the use of your sample in research, you are giving your sample without expectation of acknowledgment, compensation, interest in any commercial value or patent, or interest of any other type. However, you retain your legal rights during your participation in this research.

Will the results of research tests be reported to me?

Insert one of the following paragraphs. No. [Insert name of investigator] will use samples of your DNA only for research. The samples will not be used to plan your health care.

Note: Results given to a patient for treatment or diagnosis should be verified by a CLIA approved laboratory. If commercial testing is not available patients should consider the results of the testing investigational as described in the protocol. In addition, quality control measures should be place to avoid false positive or false negative results.

Yes. [Insert name of investigator or group] will try to get in touch with you if any results of DNA tests indicate—with high degree of certainty—that you have a risk of developing [insert name of disorder] or any other medical problem that can be treated. If you prefer that you not be contacted in the future, please make your election below:

No _____[initials]—I do not want to be contacted in the future.

Insert the next paragraph only if investigators plan to notify subjects about the results of DNA tests.

Is counseling available if I receive the results of DNA tests?

Yes. There are specialists at this medical center who can tell you what test results mean. They could make recommendations about your future plans for having children or changing habits that could affect your health.

Is there a charge for counseling?   Yes. You or your insurance provided will be responsible for the cost of the counseling.

Are there any possible benefits from receiving test results?   If you do receive the results of tests using your DNA, you may receive information that reduces the uncertainty about the likelihood of developing [insert medical problem] and/or passing it to your children.

Obtaining the results of DNA tests may help you and other members of your family plan for the future. In some cases, early treatment of a disorder that runs in the family may improve the chances of a good outcome.

What are the risks of the study?   *Insert the risk statements that are applicable to your study*
Questions

We will ask you questions about your health. However, you can skip any question that makes your uncomfortable.

Risks of blood drawing

Risks associated with drawing blood from your arm include minimal discomfort and/or bruising. Infection, excess bleeding, clotting, and/or fainting are also possible, although unlikely. If you have unusual symptoms, pain, or any other problems while you are in the study, you should report them to the researcher staff right away. Telephone numbers where they can be reached are listed on the first page of this consent form.

If blood samples are collected as part of the participants' standard medical care, please include the following sentence] You will have the same amount of blood collected whether you receive standard medical care for your health problem or take part in this research.

If blood samples are collected solely for the purpose of research, please include the following sentence. You will have *[insert amount in lay terms]* of blood collected because you are in this research study.
Sample language for a tissue repository using medical waste.

Collection of the tissue samples

Because all specimens obtained for research will come from your routinely scheduled procedures, there will be no additional risk or discomfort related to participating in this research. The only potential risk to you is accidental release of your medical information.

Stress

You could experience stress from participating in this kind of research. Knowing that researchers have personal information about you may trouble you.

*Insert the next five paragraphs **only if** subjects receive the results of DNA tests.*

If the results of DNA tests show that you or anybody else in your family may develop [insert name of disorder] or a life-threatening disease, you and other family members could experience serious stress after receiving such information.

If you experience stress because you participate in this research, [insert name of investigator or group] can help you obtain medical care to help you manage stress.

You could learn that you will not have a serious medical problem, but your children (or someone else) will.

Omit the next subsection if there is a Certificate of Confidentiality for the research project.

Problems obtaining insurance or employment

If an insurance company or employer learns that you have a high risk of developing [insert name of disorder] or a life-threatening disease, you may have problems obtaining health and/or life insurance. This could happen if you request insurance coverage for genetic or psychological counseling.

If an employer learns that you are at high risk, you may have trouble obtaining employment or being promoted. Information about you will not be released to an employer without your written permission.

Personal, sensitive information

If you are not the parent of a child in your family, or if you are the parent of a child in another family, that information could be learned from DNA tests. This kind of information will **not** be reported to you or other family members.

Unforeseen risks and new information

There may possibly be risks to your participation in this research that [Insert name of investigator] does not know about now. You will be told if any new information becomes available during the study that could cause you to change your mind about continuing to participate or that is important to your health or safety.

Loss of confidentiality   Any time information is collected, there is a potential risk of loss of confidentiality. Every effort will be made to keep your information confidential; however, this cannot be guaranteed. For more information, please see the section called "Will my information be kept confidential?"

Will I be contacted in the future?   You have the option to elect to be contacted in the future in order to obtain follow-up information or to ask you to take part in more research. (A "no" answer will not disqualify you from this research.)

    Yes _____[initials]   No _____[initials]

    If you elect "yes," please keep in touch with [insert name of investigator] and maintain a current address and telephone number on file. Please notify [insert name of investigator] if your legal name changes.

Omit the next paragraph if minors are not eligible to participate.

    It is your responsibility to inform a child that samples of his or her DNA may be kept in a research laboratory at this medical center or possibly other medical centers. The child will not be asked to sign another consent form when he/she reaches age 18.

What are the possible benefits of this study?   If you agree to take part in this study, there is usually no direct benefit to you.

    We hope the information learned from this study will benefit others with [insert condition] in the future. Information gained from this research could lead to better [insert appropriate care/prevention/treatment].

What other options do I have?   You may choose to not participate in this study. If you decide not to take part in this research study, it will have no effect on your medical care.

Will I be paid if I take part in this research study?   Yes. *Please explain what the participant will receive.*

Sample language 1:
You will be paid $100.00 at the end of the study. If you stop taking part in this study or are withdrawn by the research team, you will receive payment for only the visits you have completed. For example, if you complete four study visits you will be paid $40.00.

Sample language 2:
You will be given a $50.00 gift card to Toys R US, at the end of the study if you take part in this research.

Sample language 3:
You will be given the following, if you take part in this research:

- XYZ tote bag;
- XYZ T-shirt; and
- XYZ notepads.

Insert the following, if participant will receive a cash payment.
    If you are an employee of [insert name of host institution], your payment will be added to your regular paycheck and income tax will be deducted.
    [Insert name of host institution], as a State agency, will not be able to make any payments to you for your participation in this research if the State Comptroller has issued a "hold" on all State payments to you. Such a "hold" could result from your failure to make child support payments or pay student loans, etc. If this happens, [insert host institution] will be able to pay you for your taking part in this research (1) after you have made the outstanding payments and (2) the State Comptroller has issued a release of the "hold."
    Insert the following, if participants will receive reimbursement for travel expenses, parking, etc.
    You will be reimbursed for your parking expenses, transportation to and from the research center (e.g., cab or bus fare), or child care expenses. In order to receive reimbursement, you will need to turn in all your receipts to the research coordinator.
    *Insert the following, if participants will **not** receive reimbursement for travel expenses, parking, etc.*
    There are no funds available to pay for parking expenses, transportation to and from the research center, lost time away from work and other activities, lost wages, or child care expenses.
    If participants will not be compensated, please delete the above paragraphs and insert: No. You will not be paid to take part in this research study. There are no funds available to pay for parking expenses, transportation to and from the research center, lost time away from work and other activities, lost wages, or child care expenses.
    Insert the following, if participant will receive a cash payment and their Social Security Number will be collected.
    Your Social Security Number (SSN) will be given to [insert host institution name] in order to process your payment as required by law. This information will remain confidential unless you give your permission to share it with others, or if we are required by law to release it.

Will my insurance provider or I be charged for the costs of any part of this research study?   No. Neither you nor your insurance provider will be charged for anything done only for this research study (i.e., the Screening Procedures, Experimental Procedures, or Monitoring/Follow-up Procedures described above).

However, the expenses for routine health checkups or standard medical care for your any medical problem (care you would have received whether or not you were in this study) is your responsibility (or the responsibility of your insurance provider or governmental program). You will be charged, in the standard manner, for any procedures performed for your standard medical care.

What will happen if I am harmed as a result of taking part in this study?

It is important that you report any illness or injury to the research team listed at the top of this form immediately.

Compensation for an injury resulting from your participation in this research is not available from [insert name of host institution] or [insert other institutions, if applicable].

If applicable: The sponsor has expressed a willingness to help pay the medical expenses necessary to treat such injury.

You retain your legal rights during your participation in this research.

Will my information be kept confidential?   *Insert this section for studies without a Certificate of Confidentiality.*

Information about you that is collected for this research study will remain confidential unless you give your permission to share it with others, or if we are required by law to release it. You should know that certain organizations that may look at and/or copy your medical records for research, quality assurance, and data analysis include:

- [insert sponsor's name];
- Representatives of government agencies, like the Food and Drug Administration (FDA), involved in keeping research safe for people; and
- The [insert name of host institution] Institutional Review Board

In addition to this consent form, you will be asked to sign an "Authorization for Use and Disclosure of Protected Health Information." This authorization will give more details about how your information will be used for this research study, and who may see and/or get copies of your information.

Insert this section for studies with a Certificate of Confidentiality.

Information about you that is collected for this research study will remain confidential unless you give your permission to share it with others, or as described below. You should know that certain organizations that may look at and/or copy your medical records for research, quality assurance, and data analysis include:

- [insert sponsor's name];
- Representatives of government agencies, like the U.S. Food and Drug Administration (FDA), involved in keeping research safe for people; and
- The [insert name of host institution] Institutional Review Board.

In addition to this consent form, you will be asked to sign an "Authorization for Use and Disclosure of Protected Health Information." This authorization will give more details about how your information will be used for this research study and who may see and/or get copies of your information.

To help us further protect the information, the investigators will obtain a Certificate of Confidentiality from the U.S. Department of Health and Human Services (DHHS). This Certificate adds special protections for research information that identifies you and will help researchers protect your privacy. This Certificate does not mean the government approves or disapproves of our project.

With this Certificate of Confidentiality, the researchers cannot be forced to disclose information that may identify you in any judicial, administrative, legislative, or other proceeding, whether at the federal, state, or local level. There are situations, however, that legally require disclosure, such as:

- To DHHS for audit or program evaluation purposes;
- Information regarding test results for certain communicable diseases to the Texas Department of State Health Services, including, but not limited to HIV, hepatitis, anthrax, and smallpox;
- If you pose imminent physical harm to yourself or others;
- If you pose immediate mental or emotional injury to yourself;
- If the researchers learn that a child has been, or may be, abused or neglected; or
- If the researchers learn that an elderly or disabled person has been, or is being, abused, neglected or exploited.

The researchers will not, in any case, disclose information about you or your participation in this study unless it is included in the Authorization for Use and Disclosure of Protected Health Information for Research Purposes, or it is required by law (as mentioned above).

The Certificate of Confidentiality does not prevent you or a member of your family from voluntarily releasing information about your involvement in this research study. In addition, the researchers may not use the Certificate to withhold information about your participation in this research study if you have provided written consent to anyone allowing the researchers to release such information (including your employer or an insurance company). This means that you or your family must also actively protect your privacy.

A Certificate of Confidentiality does not represent an endorsement of this research project by the Department of Health & Human Services or any other Federal government agency.

Is there anything else I should know before I decide?

If applicable, please include:
[Insert name(s)] has/have financial interests in the company sponsoring this study. You should feel free to ask questions about this.

Whom do I call if I have questions or problems?   For questions about the study, contact [insert PI's name here] at [insert PI's number here with area code] during regular business hours and at [insert PI's 24-hour number here with area code] after hours and on weekends and holidays.

For questions about your rights as a research participant, contact the [insert name of host institution] Institutional Review Board (IRB) Office at [insert number].

SIGNATURES:

YOU WILL HAVE A COPY OF THIS CONSENT FORM TO KEEP.
Your signature below certifies the following:

- You have read (or been read) the information provided above.
- You have received answers to all of your questions and have been told who to call if you have any more questions.
- You have freely decided to participate in this research.
- You understand that you are not giving up any of your legal rights.

_____

Participant's name (printed)

_____   _____

Participant's Signature   Date

_____

Legally Authorized Representative's name (printed)

_____   _____

Legally Authorized Representative's Signature   Date

_____

Name of Person Obtaining Consent (printed)

_____   _____

Signature of Person Obtaining Consent   Date

If applicable:
ASSENT OF A MINOR:

I have discussed this research study with my parent or legal guardian and the researchers, and I agree to participate.

_____   _____

Signature of Participant (age 10 through 17)   Date

If applicable:
INTERPRETER STATEMENT:

I have interpreted this consent form into a language understandable to the participant, and the participant has agreed to participate as indicated by their signature above.

_____

Name of Interpreter (printed)

_____   _____

Signature of Interpreter   Date

Authorization for Use and Disclosure of Health Information for Research Purposes

In the document below, text denoting directions to the individual preparing the document are italicized.

Areas where text is to be added by the individual preparing the document are delineated by brackets.

NAME OF RESEARCH PARTICIPANT:

_____

Remove if not applicable.

Note: If you are a parent or guardian of a minor and have been asked to read and sign this form, the "you" in this document refers to the minor.

What is the purpose of this form?

This authorization describes how information about you and your health will be used and shared by the researcher(s) when you participate in the research study: [Abbreviated title, plus Brief description, e.g., "comparative study of two treatments for recurrent breast cancer"], to in this document as the "Research Project"). Health information is considered "protected health information" when it may directly identify you as an individual. By signing this form you are agreeing to permit the researchers and others (described in detail below) to have access to and share this information. If you have questions, please ask a member of the research team.

Who will be able to use or share my health information?

[Insert name of Institution(s)/Covered Entity(ies)] may use or share your health information with [Insert name of Principal Investigator] and his or her staff at [insert name of host institution 1] ("Researchers") for the purpose of this research study.

Will my protected health information be shared with someone other than the researchers?

Yes, the Researchers may share your health information with others who may be working with the Researchers on the Research Project ("Recipients") for purposes directly related to the conduct of this research study or as required by law. These other people or entities include:

- [Name(s) of Sponsor(s)—Delete if not applicable]. The sponsor includes any people, entities, groups or companies working for or with the sponsor, or owned by the sponsor. The sponsor will receive written reports about your participation in the research. The sponsor may look at your health information to assure the quality of the information used in the research.
- [Name(s) Collaborating Institution(s)—Delete if not applicable]. These are other research facilities that are working with [Insert name of host institution] on the Research Project.
- [Name(s) of company(ies) to supply study drug, device or resources—Delete if not applicable]. These companies are supplying the *[insert drug/device/resource]* for this study. The researchers may share your health information with these companies.
- [Name(s) of any and all outside organization(s) assisting in the research—e.g., Contract Research Organization(s), Reference Laboratories, Data Safety Monitoring Boards—Delete if not applicable]. These organizations need access to your health information to assist the Researchers in the Research Project.
- The [insert name of host institution] Institutional Review Board (IRB). This is a group of people who are responsible for assuring that the rights of participants in research are respected. Members and staff of the IRB at [Insert name of host institution] may review the records of your participation in this research. A representative of the IRB may contact you for information about your experience with this research. If you do not want to answer their questions, you may refuse to do so.
- Representatives of the Food and Drug Administration (FDA) [Delete if not applicable]. The FDA may oversee the Research Project to confirm compliance with laws and regulations. The FDA may photocopy your health information to verify information submitted to the FDA by the sponsor.
- Representatives of domestic and foreign governmental and regulatory agencies may be granted direct access to your health information for oversight, compliance activities, and determination of approval for new medicines, devices, or procedures.

How will my health information be protected?

Whenever possible your health information will be kept confidential as required by law. Federal privacy laws may not apply to other institutions, companies, or agencies collaborating with [Insert name of host institution] on this research project. [Insert name of host institution] cannot guarantee the confidentiality of your health information after it has been shared with the recipients.

Why is my personal contact information being used?

Your personal contact information is important for the [Insert name of host institution] research team to contact you during the study. However, your personal contact information will not be released without your permission.

What health information will be collected, used, and shared (disclosed)?

The Researchers will collect [List types of health information that will be collected, used, and disclosed in a way that will be meaningful to the patient. For example, type of test results, prior treatments, physical and mental history, and information collected as part of the research. Include any "sensitive" information, such as HIV status, illegal drug use, pregnancy testing, genetic testing, mental health information]. *Note: Do not list any demographic or subject contact information unless this information will be disclosed to the Recipients.*

Will my health information be used in a research report?

Yes, the research team may fill out a research report. (This is sometimes called "a case report.") The research report will not include your name, address, or telephone or social security number. The research report may include your date of birth, initials, dates you received medical care, and a tracking code. The research report will also include information the research team collects for the study.

Will my health information be used for other purposes?

Yes, the Researchers and Recipients may use your health information to create research data that do not identify you. Research data that do not identify you may be used and shared by the Researchers and Recipients in a publication about the results of the Research Project or for other research purposes not related to the Research Project.

Do I have to sign this authorization?

No, this authorization is voluntary. Your health care providers will continue to provide you with health care services even if you choose not to sign this authorization. However, if you choose not to sign this authorization, you cannot take part in this Research Project.

How long will my permission last?

This authorization has no expiration date. You may cancel this authorization at any time. If you decide to cancel this authorization, you will no longer be able to take part in the Research Project. The researchers may still use and share the health information that they have already collected before you canceled the authorization. To cancel this authorization, you must make this request in writing to: [Principal Investigator or Designee, address, and phone number].

Will I receive a copy of this authorization?

Yes, a copy of this authorization will be provided to you.

SIGNATURES:

By signing this document you are permitting [Insert name of host institution] to use and disclose health information about you for research purposes as described above.

_____   _____
Signature of Research Participant   Date

For Legal Representatives of Research Participants (if applicable):

Printed Name of Legal Representative: _____

Relationship to Research Participant: _____

I certify that I have the legal authority under applicable law to make this authorization on behalf of the Research Participant identified above. The basis for this legal authority is:

_____

(e.g., parent, legal guardian, person with legal power of attorney, etc.)

_____   _____
Signature of legal representative   Date

Combined Template for Informed Consent and HIPAA Authorization

In the document below, text denoting directions to the individual preparing the document are italicized.

Areas where text is to be added by the individual preparing the document are delineated by brackets.

[Institutions where research is to be conducted]

CONSENT TO PARTICIPATE IN RESEARCH

Title of Research: [insert title]

Funding Agency / Sponsor: [if no external funds, state source of support]

Insert the names of the investigators and those individuals who will obtain consent.

Study Doctors: [insert investigators names]

Research Personnel: [insert research personnel names]

You may call these study doctors or research personnel during regular office hours at [insert phone number]. At other times, you may call them at [insert after hours phone number].

Remove if not applicable.

Note: If you are a parent or guardian of a minor and have been asked to read and sign this form, the "you" in this document refers to the minor.

Instructions

Please read this consent form carefully and take your time making a decision about whether to participate. As the researchers discuss this consent form with you, please ask him/her to explain any words or information that you do not clearly understand. The purpose of the study, risks, inconveniences, discomforts, and other important information about the study are listed below. If you decide to participate, you will be given a copy of this form to keep.

Why is this study being done?

This study is being done to [please complete]. *Sample language—The study is being done to find out whether an investigational (non-FDA approved) drug called [insert drug name] can treat your condition better or more safely than standard medication.*

Please note: If you are using an investigational drug, drug combination, and/or device, please always indicate what is FDA approved and what is investigational, and define "investigational." For example: "The word 'investigational' means the [insert study drug or device or biologic] is still being tested in research studies and is not approved by the U.S. Food and Drug Administration (FDA)." Refrain from using "medicine," "treatment," or "therapy" for the investigational drug or device. Instead, use "study drug," "study procedures," "study processes," etc.

Why is this considered research?

This is a research study because [complete this sentence, assuring that all experimental or investigational drugs, devices, and/or procedures are clearly identified and defined].

Sample phrases for unapproved drugs, devices, or procedures:

- *[Insert drug/device name] is investigational and has not been approved by the U.S. Food and Drug Administration (FDA) for the treatment of [insert disease or condition].*
- *[Insert drug/device name] has been approved by the FDA to treat [insert approved use].*
- *[Insert drug name] is being compared to a standard drug, [insert standard drug name], that has already been approved by the FDA. The researchers are interested in learning which drug is more effective and/or safer in treating your condition/disorder.*
- *[Insert procedure] is being compared to the standard procedure [insert procedure here]. The researchers are interested in learning which procedure is more effective and/or safer in treating your condition/disorder.*

The following definitions may help you understand this study: *Delete definitions that do not apply to this study.*

- Double-blind means neither you nor the researchers will know which [insert applicable term: drug or device] you are receiving.
- Placebo controlled means that some participants will get a placebo. A placebo looks like the investigational drug but it includes no active ingredients (e.g., a sugar pill).
- Randomization means you will be placed by chance (like a flip of a coin) in one of the study groups. For studies with more than two arms, use "like drawing straws" instead of "flip of a coin."
- Single-blind means that you will not know which [insert applicable term: drug or device] you are receiving but the researchers will know.
- Standard medical care means the regular care you would receive from your personal doctor if you choose not to participate in this research.
- Researchers mean the study doctor and research personnel at [insert names of institutions from which patients will be recruited] and its affiliated hospitals.

Why am I being asked to take part in this research study?

You are being asked to take part in this study because [outline briefly the reason this study is being conducted].

Sample language:
You are being asked to take part in this study because you have high blood pressure.

Do I have to take part in this research study?

No. You have the right to choose whether you want to take part in this research study. If you decide to participate and later change your mind, you are free to stop participation at any time.

If you decide not to take part in this research study it will not change your legal rights or the quality of health care that you receive at this center.

How many people will take part in this study?

About [insert number] people will take part in this study at [insert names of institutions from which patients will be recruited]. *If a multicenter trial, please also insert: "This study also is taking place at a number of other medical facilities around the country. There will be a total of [insert number] people participating in this research study throughout the United States and / or other countries."*

What is involved in the study?

If you volunteer to take part in this research study, you will be asked to sign this consent form and will have the following tests and procedures. Some of the procedures may be part of your standard medical care, but others are being done solely for the purpose of this study.

Screening procedures   To help decide if you qualify to be in this study, the researchers may ask you questions about your health, including medications you take and any surgical procedures you have had.

You may also have to fill out certain forms or have the following examinations, tests, or procedures:

Sample language:

- *Physical examination and medical history;*
- *Vital signs;*
- *Blood tests;*
- *Electrocardiogram (EKG), a tracing of the electrical activity of the heart; and*
- *Demographic information (age, sex, ethnic origin).*

If applicable:

Group assignment   If the researchers believe you can take part in this study, you will be assigned randomly (like a flip of a coin) to receive either [insert study drug or procedure] or [insert placebo (inactive substance) or other study arm]. You have a [insert number] in [insert number] chance of receiving [insert name of the medication, device procedure, etc.] or placebo. *For studies with more than two arms, use "like drawing straws" instead of "flipping a coin."*

If applicable:

The group you will be in is decided by [insert who determines the randomization]. Neither you nor the researchers will be allowed to choose which group you are assigned to.

If the study is not blinded, please delete the following paragraph:

Neither you nor the researchers will know which group you are in. However, the sponsor will release the information about your assignment to the researchers if it is needed for your safety.

If applicable:

Study medication/intervention   [Insert description of the study medication or study intervention].

For example:

If you decide to participate in this study you will take either:

- *1 tablet of alpha-peg (10 mg) twice a day or*
- *1 tablet of pegatron (25 mg) twice a day*

Procedures and evaluations during the research   *Explain the procedures and evaluations (as outlined in the protocol). Clearly identify any inconvenient, experimental, or painful procedures (such as long clinic visits, keeping a detailed diary between clinic visits, collection of multiple blood samples, etc.)*

Specify the amount of blood that will be drawn at any one time in teaspoons, tablespoons, or cups.

Specify the number of study visits and the approximate length of time it will take to complete each study visit.

When describing what is involved in the study, please consider using a detailed timeline.

For example:

You will have the following tests and/or evaluations:

Visit 1:

- *Physical examination;*
- *An EKG; and*
- *Two tablespoons of blood will be drawn from your arm by needle stick for blood tests.*

Visit 2:

- *You will receive the study drug intravenously (into your vein) for 2 hours and*
- *You will complete two questionnaires.*

Or insert a simple table

The [insert research-related test(s)] in this study are designed for research, not for medical purposes. They are not useful for finding problems or diseases. Even though the researchers are not looking at your [insert research-related test(s)] to find or treat a medical problem, you will be told if they notice something unusual. You and your regular doctor can decide together whether to follow up with more tests or treatment. Because the [insert research-related test(s)] done in this study are not for medical purposes, the research results will not be sent to you or to your regular doctor.

Procedures for storing of extra or leftover samples   *Please note if DNA testing will be completed on the samples, a separate DNA Consent Form must be completed.*

Explain the procedures for the storing of the extra or leftover samples and the purpose of storing the samples. This information should include:

- *How the samples will be labeled;*
- *Whether or not identifiers will be kept;*
- *Location of where the samples will be kept; and*
- *Who will have access to the samples?*

Insert the following, if the study will collect and use the subject's social security number.

The researchers will record and use your Social Security Number (SSN) in order to [state intended use]. You do not have to give this information to the researchers; however, it may result in [state what may happen if the subject fails to provide SSN]. This information will remain confidential unless you give your permission to share it with others or if we are required by law to release it.

How long can I expect to be in this study?

Please describe here how long the study will be (in weeks, days, or months). Describe also (if applicable) whether you intend to collect follow-up information, and how much time that collection will require. For example, until 6 months after last study drug dose, for the rest of your life, etc.]

You can choose to stop participating for any reason at any time. However, if you decide to stop participating in the study, we encourage you to tell the researchers. You may be asked if you are willing to complete some study termination tests.

What are the risks of the study?

Please note: The risk section should only contain the risks associated with study procedures. Risks of standard medical care procedures that are not required for this study should not be included in the consent form.

Please list only the risks and side effects related to the investigational aspects of the study and any standard of care procedures that are mandated for entry and during the course of the study. Any risks from standard medical care procedures that are not specially mandated should not be included.

For example: A patient who is undergoing joint replacement surgery for osteoarthritis, and the surgeon wants to participate in a trial of a new postoperative analgesic. The risks of the general anesthesia or orthopedic surgery do not need to be included in the Consent Form. However, for a trial of a drug-eluting stents versus medical management, all of the risks regarding the stent procedure would need to be included even though the procedure is standard of care.

Study procedure/intervention   Because of your participation in this study, you are at risk for the following side effects. You should discuss these with the researchers and your regular health care provider.

[Insert study drug name] may cause some, all or none of the side effects listed below.

Please list only the risks and side effects related to the investigational aspects of the study, and do not list side effects of supportive medications unless the medications are specifically mandated by the study.

Please insert a separate section for each study drug / device / procedure. Please include the frequency of the side effects in percentages. Large ranges, such as "2% to 60%" should be avoided. Since there is no standard definition of frequent, occasional, or rare, as a guide, "frequent" can be viewed as occurring in greater than 20% of subjects, "occasional" as 2% to 20% of subjects, and "rare" as less than 2% of subjects. However, frequencies may be adapted to specific study agents. If more specific data are not available, use the largest percent.

For example:

	Frequent (30% of subjects)	Occasional (15% of subjects)	Rare (less than 1% of subjects)
Serious		*Blood clots in lungs*	*Death*
			Irregular heart beat
Less serious	*Low white blood cells*	*Moderate rash*	*Itching*
Minor	*Headache*	*Mild rash*	*Hiccups*
		Trouble sleeping	

or

Frequent	Occasionally
• *Headache*	• *Blood clots in lungs*
• *Trouble sleeping*	• *Moderate rash*
Rare	*Serious but rare*
• *Hiccups*	• *Death*
	• *Irregular heart beat*

Psychological stress   *If the study involves psychological stress, please state.* Some of the questions we will ask you as part of this study may make you feel uncomfortable. You may refuse to answer any of the questions, take a break, or stop your participation in this study at any time.

Loss of confidentiality   Any time information is collected; there is a potential risk for loss of confidentiality. Every effort will be made to keep your information confidential; however, this cannot be guaranteed.

Please note: For class D medications please use the risk to an embryo or fetus language provided by the sponsor and the FDA instead of, or in addition to, the following template language in the "Risks to Sperm, Embryo, Fetus, or Breast-Fed Infant" section.

Risks to sperm, embryo, fetus, or breast-fed infant

Males: Being in this research may damage your sperm, which could cause harm to a child that you may father while on this study. If you take part in this study and are sexually active, you must agree to use a medically acceptable form of birth control. Medically acceptable forms of birth control include:

(1) Surgical sterilization (vasectomy) or

(2) A condom used with a spermicide (a substance that kills sperm).

Females: If you are part of this study while pregnant or breast-feeding an infant, it is possible that you may expose the unborn child or infant to risks. For that reason, pregnant and breast-feeding females cannot participate in the study. If you can become pregnant, a blood pregnancy test will be done (using one teaspoon of blood drawn from a vein by needle stick), and it must be negative before you participate in this study. If you take part in this study and you are sexually active, you and any person that you have sex with must use medically acceptable birth control (contraceptives) during the study. Medically acceptable birth control (contraceptives) includes:

(1) Surgical sterilization (such as hysterectomy or "tubes tied"),
(2) Approved hormonal contraceptives (such as birth control pills, patch, or ring; Depo-Provera, Depo-Lupron, Implanon),
(3) Barrier methods (such as condom or diaphragm) used with a spermicide (a substance that kills sperm), or
(4) An intrauterine device (IUD).

If you do become pregnant during this study, you must tell the researchers immediately.

If the study will include exposure to radiation, please include the following:
Radiation exposure to a woman's reproductive organs may harm an embryo or fetus. Also, if radioactive materials are used for certain types of scans, harm may come to an embryo, fetus, or an infant who is breast-feeding.

Pregnancy tests performed during the early stages of pregnancy do not always reveal pregnancy. Therefore, radiation exposure that includes the reproductive organs will be limited to the first 10 days after a woman who can become pregnant (age 10 to 50 years) has begun her most recent menstrual period. This is a standard policy in clinics and hospitals within [insert names of institutions from which patients will be recruited]. This policy applies unless there is an important medical reason requiring radiation outside this time frame.

If minors will be enrolled in the study, please insert the following:
If your parents or guardian asks, we will tell them the results of your pregnancy test or that you are using birth control.

Risks of radiation—diagnostic test   *Insert the risk statement if applicable to your study.*

If the amount of radiation exposure is the same regardless as to whether the participant elects to participate in this research study or receives standard medical care, please include the following sentence. The radiation dose that you will get from diagnostic tests is medically indicated for your condition, and it is the same that you would get if you were not involved in this research study.

If the amount of radiation exposure is more than the participant would receive if they elected to receive standard medical care, please include one of the following sentences.

If additional radiation dose < 350 mrem from research:
This research study includes exposure to radiation from diagnostic tests in addition to radiation that you would receive from standard care. The additional radiation dose you will get is about [insert percentage] % of the average radiation dose from all sources (natural background radiation, consumer appliances, radon gas, medical tests, etc.) that a person in the United States receives each year. (The exact wording and estimate should be defined by consultation with local [insert name of institution] Radiation Safety Committee or equivalent administrative office.)

If additional radiation dose > 350 mrem from research:

This research study includes exposure to radiation from diagnostic tests in addition to that you would receive from standard care. The risk of harm to your body from this radiation can be compared to risks from everyday activities. For example, the risk of developing fatal cancer during your lifetime from this radiation is comparative to the risk of suffering a fatal car crash while driving [XX] miles in an automobile. The average household in the United States drives 23,000 miles per year (2001 data). (The exact wording and estimate should be defined by consultation with local [institutional] Radiation Safety Committee or equivalent administrative office.)

If additional radiation dose involving cardiac catheterization, electrophysiology studies, and interventional peripheral and neuroradiology procedures, the investigator should consult with a medical physicist to determine if additional statements covering any deterministic effects—such as erythema or epilation—may be required.

Risks of radiation—radiation therapy   *If the amount of radiation exposure is the same regardless as to whether the participant elects to participate in this research study or receives standard medical care, please include the following text.*

The radiation therapy used in this research is the standard radiation therapy for your health problem; therefore, the risk of harm to your body is the same. Your radiation doctor will discuss the known risks of radiation therapy with you and ask you to sign a separate specific treatment site consent form.

High-dose radiation treatments to or near a man's testicles or a woman's ovaries may produce harmful changes that could be passed on to children through a sperm or an egg.

Women: Females (ages 10 to 50 years) able to have children should avoid becoming pregnant until after they have had three menstrual periods after the end of all radiation therapy. After three menstrual periods, there is almost no risk of harmful changes to an egg.

Men: Males must avoid fathering a child until 10 weeks after the end of all radiation therapy. After that period, there is much less risk of harmful changes to sperm. Even then there is still an unknown amount of risk.

Possible side effects of radiation therapy to the (site) include: (select the appropriate short- and long-term effects from risk information that will be available by consultation with the local [institutional] Radiation Safety Committee. The exact wording and estimate should be defined by consultation with this committee).

If the amount of radiation exposure is different from the standard of care, please include the following sentence.

The radiation therapy in this research is different from the standard radiation therapy for your health problem. The radiation dose that will be used is (more/less/given in a different way) than the standard treatment. The potential risks of this dose include: [consult with radiation oncologist for assistance].

Risks of blood drawing   *Insert the risk statement if applicable to your study*

Risks associated with drawing blood from your arm include minimal discomfort and/or bruising. Infection, excess bleeding, clotting, and/or fainting also are possible, although unlikely.

If blood samples are collected as part of the participants' standard medical care, please include the following sentence. You will have the same amount of blood collected whether you receive standard medical care for your health problem or take part in this research.

If blood samples are collected solely for the purpose of research, please include the following sentence. You will have [insert amount in lay terms] of blood collected because you are in this research study.

If applicable:

Placebo   If you receive a placebo, you will not receive active medication for your health problem. If your problem becomes worse, your participation in the research will stop. If this happens, your study doctor can discuss alternative care with you.

Note: The amount of blood that can be collected may differ from institution to institution and is defined locally by individual IRBs. In adults, this is a relatively large volume and may be modified by the presence of anemia or other intercurrent illnesses. In the pediatric age groups, this quantity is more restricted and varies by age and weight. These volumes and frequencies should be obtained from the local institutional IRB office.

Other risks   There may possibly be other side effects that are unknown at this time. If you are concerned about other, unknown side effects, please discuss this with the researchers.

How will risks be minimized or prevented?

Describe how the study design and procedures will prevent and/or minimize any potential risks or discomfort. Potential risks and discomforts must be minimized to the greatest extent possible by using procedures such as appropriate training of personnel, monitoring, or withdrawal of the subject upon evidence of difficulty or adverse event and referral for treatment, counseling or other necessary follow-up.

What will my responsibilities be during the study?

While you are part of this study, the researchers will follow you closely to determine whether there are problems that need medical care. It is your responsibility to do the following:

- Ask questions about anything you do not understand.
- Keep your appointments.
- Follow the researchers' instructions.
- Let the researchers know if your telephone number or address changes.
- Store study materials [insert tablets, vials of liquid, needles, etc. as applicable] in a secure place at home away from anyone who is unable to read and understand labels, especially children.
- Tell the researchers before you take any new medication, even if it is prescribed by another doctor for a different medical problem or something purchased over the counter.
- Tell your regular doctor about your participation in this study.
- If study involves medication, please state. Carry information about [the research medication] in your purse or wallet.
- Report to the researchers any injury or illnesses while you are on study even if you do not think it is related.

If I agree to take part in this research study, will I be told of any new risks that may be found during the course of the study?

Yes. You will be told if any new information becomes available during the study that could cause you to change your mind about continuing to participate or that is important to your health or safety.

What should I do if I think I am having problems?

If you have unusual symptoms, pain, or any other problems while you are in the study, you should report them to the researchers right away. Telephone numbers where they can be reached are listed on the first page of this consent form.

If you have a sudden, serious problem, like difficulty breathing or severe pain, go to the nearest hospital emergency room, or call 911 (or the correct emergency telephone number in your area). Tell emergency personnel about any medications you are taking, including any medications you are taking for this study.

What are the possible benefits of this study?

Please note: The description of benefits to the participant should be clear and not overstated. If no direct benefit is anticipated, then that should be stated. If these benefits may be materially relevant to a participant's decision to participate, the benefits should be disclosed in the informed consent document.

If you agree to take part in this study, there [may or may not] be direct benefits to you. The researchers cannot guarantee that you will benefit from participation in this research.

We hope the information learned from this study will benefit others with [insert condition] in the future. Information gained from this research could lead to better [insert appropriate term, such as 'care', 'prevention', or 'treatment'].

What options are available if I decide not to take part in this research study?

If a treatment study, insert: You do not have to participate in this research to receive care for your medical problem. Instead of being in this study, you have the following options:

- [Please insert all alternative treatment options available to the participant] *Please note: when applicable, this should include receiving the study drug or treatment off study or the possibility of no treatment at all.*

Please talk to the researchers or your personal doctor about these options.

If not a treatment study, insert: This is not a treatment study. You do not have to be part of it to get treatment for your condition.

Will I be paid if I take part in this research study?

Yes. *Please explain what the participant will receive.*

Sample language 1:

You will be paid $100.00 at the end of the study. If you stop taking part in this study or are withdrawn by the research team, you will receive payment for only the visits you have completed. For example, if you complete four study visits you will be paid $40.00.

Sample language 2:

You will be given a $50.00 gift card to Toys R US at the end of the study if you take part in this research.

Sample language 3:

You will be given the following, if you take part in this research:

- *XYZ tote bag;*
- *XYZ T-shirt; and*
- *XYZ notepads.*

If applicable:

There are no funds available to pay for parking expenses, transportation to and from the research center, lost time away from work and other activities, lost wages, or child care expenses.

Insert the following, if participant will receive a cash payment and their social security number will be collected.

Your Social Security Number (SSN) will be given to [insert name of host institution] in order to process your payment as required by law. This information will remain confidential unless you give your permission to share it with others, or if we are required by law to release it.

Insert the following, if participant will receive a cash payment.

If you are an employee of [insert name of host institution], your payment will be added to your regular paycheck and income tax will be deducted.

If applicable:

[insert name of host institution], as a State agency, will not be able to make any payments to you for your participation in this research if the State Comptroller has issued a "hold" on all State payments to you. Such a "hold" could result from your failure to make child support payments, pay student loans, etc. If this happens, [insert name of host institution] will be able to pay you for your taking part in this research (1) after you have made the outstanding payments and (2) the State Comptroller has issued a release of the "hold."

Insert the following, if participants will receive reimbursement for travel expenses, parking, etc.

You will be reimbursed for your parking expenses, transportation to and from the research center (e.g., cab or bus fare), or child care expenses. In order to receive reimbursement, you will need to turn in all your receipts to the research coordinator.

If participants will not be compensated, please delete the above paragraphs and insert: No. You will not be paid to take part in this research study. There are no funds available to pay for parking expenses, transportation to and from the research center, lost time away from work and other activities, lost wages, or child care expenses.

Will my insurance provider or I be charged for the costs of any part of this research study?

No. Neither you nor your insurance provider will be charged for anything done only for this research study (i.e., the Screening Procedures, Experimental Procedures, or Monitoring/Follow-up Procedures described above).

However, the standard medical care for your condition (care you would have received whether or not you were in this study) is your responsibility (or the responsibility of your insurance provider or governmental program). You will be charged, in the standard manner, for any procedures performed for your standard medical care.

Please note: If the participant's insurance company will be responsible for any research-related costs, please use the following language:

Yes. The costs of [insert items] will be billed to you or your insurance provider. We expect the costs of [insert items] to be [insert amount].

What will happen if I am harmed as a result of taking part in this study?

It is important that you report any illness or injury to the research team listed at the top of this form immediately.

Compensation for an injury resulting from your participation in this research is not available from [insert name of host institution] or [insert other institutions, if applicable].

If applicable: The sponsor has expressed a willingness to help pay the medical expenses necessary to treat such injury.

You retain your legal rights during your participation in this research.

Can I stop taking part in this research study?

Yes. If you decide to participate and later change your mind, you are free to stop taking part in the research study at any time.

If you decide to stop taking part in this research study, it will not affect your relationship with the [insert name of host institution] staff or doctors. Whether you participate or not will have no effect on your legal rights or the quality of your health care.

If you are a medical student, fellow, faculty, or staff at [insert name of host institution], your status will not be affected in any way.

Include if recruiting from investigator's own patients:

Your doctor is a research investigator in this study. S/he is interested in both your medical care and the conduct of this research study. At any time, you may discuss your care with another doctor who is not part of this research study. You do not have to take part in any research study offered by your doctor.

If I agree to take part in this research study, can I be removed from the study without my consent?

Yes. The researchers may decide to take you off this study if:

- Your medical problem remains unchanged or becomes worse.
- The researchers believe that participation in the research is no longer safe for you.
- The researchers believe that other treatment may be more helpful.
- The sponsor or the FDA stops the research for the safety of the participants.
- The sponsor cancels the research.
- You are unable to keep appointments or to follow the researcher's instructions.

Will my information be kept confidential?

Insert this section for studies without a Certificate of Confidentiality.

Information about you that is collected for this research study will remain confidential unless you give your permission to share it with others, or if we are required by law to release it. We know that this information is private. The federal privacy regulations of the Health Insurance Portability and Accountability Act (HIPAA) protect your identifiable health information. If you authorize us to use your information, we will protect it as required by law.

Insert this section for studies without a Certificate of Confidentiality.

By signing this form, you are permitting [Name of Institution(s)/Covered Entity(ies)] to use or share your health information with [Name of Principal Investigator] and his or her staff at [insert name of host institution] ("Researchers") for the purpose of this research study.

Insert this section for studies with a Certificate of Confidentiality.

Information about you that is collected for this research study will remain confidential unless you give your permission to share it with others, or if we are required by law to release it. We know that this information is private. The federal privacy regulations of the Health Insurance Portability and Accountability Act (HIPAA) protect your identifiable health information. If you authorize us to use your information we will protect it as required by law.

By signing this form, you are permitting [Name of Institution(s)/Covered Entity(ies)] to use or share your health information with [Name of Principal Investigator] and his or her staff at [insert name of host institution] ("Researchers") for the purpose of this research study.

To help us further protect the information, the investigators will obtain a Certificate of Confidentiality from the U.S. Department of Health and Human Services (DHHS). This Certificate adds special protections for research information that identifies you and will help researchers protect your privacy.

With this Certificate of Confidentiality, the researchers cannot be forced to disclose information that may identify you in any judicial, administrative, legislative, or other proceeding, whether at the federal, state, or local level. There are situations, however, where we will voluntarily disclose information consistent with state or other laws, such as:

- To DHHS for audit or program evaluation purposes;
- Information regarding test results for certain communicable diseases to the Texas Department of State Health Services, including, but not limited to HIV, hepatitis, anthrax, and smallpox;
- If you pose imminent physical harm to yourself or others;
- If you pose immediate mental or emotional injury to yourself;
- If the researchers learn that a child has been, or may be, abused or neglected; or
- If the researchers learn that an elderly or disabled person has been, or is being, abused, neglected or exploited.

The researchers will not, in any case, disclose information about you or your participation in this study unless it is included in the Authorization for Use and Disclosure of Protected Health Information for Research Purposes as stated above.

The Certificate of Confidentiality does not prevent you or a member of your family from voluntarily releasing information about your involvement in this research study. In addition, the researchers may not use the Certificate to withhold information about your participation in this research study if you have provided written consent to anyone allowing the researchers to release such information (including your employer or an insurance company). This means that you or your family must also actively protect your privacy.

A Certificate of Confidentiality does not represent an endorsement of this research project by the Department of Health & Human Services or any other Federal government agency.

Will my protected health information be shared with someone other than the researchers?

Yes, the Researchers may share your health information with others who may be working with the Researchers on the Research Project ("Recipients") for purposes directly related to the conduct of this research study or as required by law. These other people or entities include:

- [Name(s) of Sponsor(s) - Delete if not applicable]. The sponsor includes any people, entities, groups or companies working for or with the sponsor, or owned by the sponsor. The sponsor will receive written reports about your participation in the research. The sponsor may look at your health information to assure the quality of the information used in the research.
- [Name(s) Collaborating Institution(s) - Delete if not applicable]. These are other research facilities that are working with [insert name of host institution] on the Research Project.
- [Name(s) of company(ies) to supply study drug, device or resources - Delete if not applicable]. These companies are supplying the *[insert drug / device / resource]* for this study. The Researchers may share your health information with these companies.
- [Name(s) of any and all outside organization(s) assisting in the research—e.g., Contract Research Organization(s), Reference Laboratories, Data Safety Monitoring Boards - Delete if not applicable]. These organizations need access to your health information to assist the Researchers in the Research Project.
- The [insert name of host institution] Institutional Review Board (IRB). This is a group of people who are responsible for assuring that the rights of participants in research are respected. Members and staff of the IRB at [insert name of host institution] may review the records of your participation in this research. A representative of the IRB may contact you for information about your experience with this research. If you do not want to answer their questions, you may refuse to do so.
- Representatives of the Food and Drug Administration (FDA) [Delete if not applicable]. The FDA may oversee the Research Project to confirm compliance with laws and regulations. The FDA may photocopy your health information to verify information submitted to the FDA by the sponsor.
- Representatives of domestic and foreign governmental and regulatory agencies may be granted direct access to your health information for oversight, compliance activities, and determination of approval for new medicines, devices, or procedures.

What health information will be collected, used, and shared (disclosed)?

The Researchers will collect [List types of health information that will be collected, used, and disclosed in a way that will be meaningful to the patient. For example, type of test results, prior treatments, physical and mental history, and information collected as part of the research. Include any "sensitive" information, such as HIV status, illegal drug use, pregnancy testing, genetic testing, mental health information].

Will my health information be used for other purposes?

Yes, the Researchers and Recipients may use your health information to create research data that do not identify you. Research data that do not identify you may be used and shared by the Researchers and Recipients in a publication about the results of the Research Project or for other research purposes not related to the Research Project.

How long will my permission last?

This authorization has no expiration date. You may cancel this authorization at any time. If you decide to cancel this authorization, you will no longer be able to take part in the Research Project. The researchers may still use and share the health information that they have already collected before you canceled the authorization. To cancel this authorization, you must make this request in writing to: [Principal Investigator or Designee, address, and phone number].

Are there procedures I should follow after stopping participation in this research?

Include this section if there are procedures to be followed or risks to participants after stopping participation in the research study.

Please specify what a participant will be asked to do in the event of early withdrawal from the study. Identify any materials (study pills, injections, liquids, creams, etc.) that need to be returned.

If applicable, please explain that sudden discontinuation of the study medication (such as corticosteroids or antipsychotic medications) or study device could be unsafe.

For example:

Yes. If you, the researchers, or the sponsor stops your participation in the research, you may be asked to do the following:

- *Let the researchers know immediately that you wish to withdraw from the research.*
- *Return to the research center for tests that may be needed for your safety.*
- *Return any unused study materials, including empty containers.*
- *Discuss your future medical care, if any, with the researchers and / or your personal doctor.*

If applicable, please include:

Is there anything else I should know before I decide?

[Insert name(s)] has/have financial interests in the company sponsoring this study. You should feel free to ask questions about this.

Whom do I call if I have questions or problems?

For questions about the study, contact [insert PI's name here] at [insert PI's number here with area code] during regular business hours and at [insert PI's 24-hour number here with area code] after hours and on weekends and holidays.

For questions about your rights as a research participant, contact the [insert name of host institution] Institutional Review Board (IRB) Office at xxx-xxx-xxxx.

SIGNATURES:

YOU WILL BE GIVEN A COPY OF THIS CONSENT FORM TO KEEP
Your signature below certifies the following:

- You have read (or been read) the information provided above.
- You have received answers to all of your questions and have been told who to call if you have any more questions.

- You have freely decided to participate in this research.
- You understand that you are not giving up any of your legal rights.

_____

Participant's Name (printed)

_____   _____

Participant's Signature   Date

_____

Legally Authorized Representative's Name (printed)

_____   _____

Legally Authorized Representative's Signature   Date

_____

Name of person obtaining consent (printed)

_____   _____

Signature of person obtaining consent   Date

If applicable:
ASSENT OF A MINOR:

I have discussed this research study with my parent or legal guardian and the researchers, and I agree to participate.

_____   _____

Signature of participant (age 10 through 17)   Date

If applicable:
INTERPRETER STATEMENT:

I have interpreted this consent form into a language understandable to the participant, and the participant has agreed to participate as indicated by their signature on the associated short form.

_____

Name of interpreter (printed)

_____   _____

Signature of interpreter   Date

Request for Waiver of HIPAA Privacy Authorization for Research

[INSERT INSTITUTION NAME]

Request for Waiver of HIPAA Privacy Authorization for Research

IRB Number: _____

Study Title: _____

Principal Investigator: _____

Principal Investigator Mail Code: _____

Research Coordinator: _____

Research Coordinator Phone #: _____

Research Coordinator Mail Code / Address
  (if applicable): _____

SEE INSTRUCTION PAGE FOR GUIDANCE AND EXAMPLES

1. I am requesting this waiver of authorization for the following purpose:

   Please select only one

   ❑ The collection of initial screening data to recruit potential research subjects, or to determine study eligibility only. (Authorization is required for the remainder of the research study.)

   ❑ Retrospective reviews, research database or repository, or other research study where obtaining a signed authorization is not practical.

2. The following protected health information will be created, collected, used and/or disclosed for the purpose of conducting this research: *(Please list the specific protected health information that will be sought under this waiver)*

3. I certify that the use or disclosure of protected health information involves no more than minimal risk to the privacy of individuals based on at least the following elements:

   a. An adequate plan is in place to protect the identifiers from improper use and disclosure. The plan is as follows:

Select all that apply. Include additional information when applicable.

❑ All electronic study data will be password protected.
❑ Passwords will be changed on a regular basis.
❑ Access to study data will be restricted to the following authorized study personnel only.

_____

_____

_____

❑ All paper study records will be kept in locked file cabinets and access limited to authorized study personnel only.
❑ Other:_____

_____

_____

b. An adequate plan is in place to destroy the identifiers at the earliest opportunity consistent with conduct of the research, unless there is a health or research justification for retaining the identifiers or such retention is otherwise required by law. The plan is as follows:

c. The protected health information will not be reused or disclosed to any other person or entity, except as required by law, for authorized oversight of the research study, or for other research for which the use or disclosure of protected health information would be permitted by HIPAA regulations.

4. I certify that the research could not practicably be conducted without this requested waiver.

5. I certify that this research could not practicably be conducted without access to and use of the protected health information.

6. I certify that I will only access the minimum amount of protected health information necessary to accomplish the purpose(s) of the research described under this waiver.

I attest that the above statements are correct and complete to the best of my knowledge.

_____   _____
Signature of Principal Investigator   Date

_____
Printed name of Principal Investigator

FOR IRB OFFICE USE ONLY

This waiver was   Full Review   Expedited Review
    approved under: _____   _____
                               Signature of IRB Administrative   Approval Date
                               Representative or Board Member

National Institutes of Health (NIH) Application for a Public Health Service Grant Form PHS 398 Definition of Direct Costs

Personnel

Name. Starting with the PD/PI(s), list the names of all applicant organization employees who are involved on the project during the initial budget period, regardless of whether a salary is requested. Include all collaborating investigators, individuals in training, and support staff.

Role on Project. Identify the role of each individual listed on the project. Describe their specific functions under Justification on Form Page 5. Provide budget narrative for ALL personnel by position, role, and level of effort using person months (calendar, academic and/or summer). This includes any "to-be-appointed" positions.

Months Devoted to Project. Enter the number of months devoted to the project. Three columns are provided depending on the type of appointment being reflected: academic, calendar, and/or summer months. Individuals may have consecutive appointments within a calendar year, for example, for an academic period and a summer period. In this case, each appointment should be identified separately using the corresponding column.

If effort does not change throughout the year, use only the calendar months column. If effort varies between academic and summer months, leave the calendar months column blank and use only the academic and summer months columns. In cases where no contractual appointment exists with the applicant organization and salary is requested, enter the number of months for the requested period.

Institutional Base Salary. An applicant organization may choose to leave this column blank. However, PHS staff will require this information prior to award. See Definitions in Part III.3.

Salary Requested. Regardless of the number of months being devoted to the project, indicate only the amount of salary being requested for this budget period for each individual listed.

Some PHS grant programs are currently subject to a legislatively imposed salary limitation. Any adjustment for salary limits will be made at the time of award. For guidance on current salary limitations see the *Salary Cap Summary* on the NIH grants Web site or contact the organization's office of sponsored programs.

NIH grants also limit the compensation for graduate students. Compensation includes salary or wages, fringe benefits, and tuition remission. While actual institutional-based compensation should be requested and justified, this may be adjusted at the time of the award. For more guidance on this policy, see: http://grants.nih.gov/grants/guide/notice-files/NOT-OD-02-017.html.

Fringe Benefits. Fringe benefits may be requested in accordance with institutional guidelines for each position, provided the costs are treated consistently by the applicant organization as a direct cost to all sponsors.

Totals. Calculate the totals for each position and enter the subtotals in each column where indicated.

The applicant organization and its consortium/contractor(s) may omit salaries and fringe benefits for individuals from copies of the application that are available to non-Federal reviewers. In such cases, replace the numbers with asterisks. You must show the subtotals. Provide one copy, for use only by PHS staff, with the asterisks replaced by the salaries and fringe benefits.

Special instructions for joint university and department of veterans affairs (VA) appointments

Individuals with joint university and VA appointments may request the university's share of their salary in proportion to the effort devoted to the research project. The individual's salary with the university determines the base for computing that request. Signature by the institutional official on the application certifies that: (1) the individual is applying as part of a joint appointment specified by a formal Memorandum of Understanding between the university and the VA and (2) there is no possibility of dual compensation for the same work, or of an actual or apparent conflict of interest regarding such work. Additional information may be requested by the awarding components.

Consultant costs

Whether or not costs are involved, provide the names and organizational affiliations of all consultants, other than those involved in consortium/contractual arrangements. Include consultant physicians in connection with patient care and persons who are confirmed to serve on external monitoring or advisory committees. Describe the services to be performed on Form Page 5 under "Justification." Include the number of days of anticipated consultation, the expected rate of compensation, travel, per diem, and other related costs.

Equipment

List each item of equipment with amount requested separately and justify each purchase on Form Page 5.

Supplies

Itemize supplies in separate categories, such as glassware, chemicals, radioisotopes, etc. Categories in amounts less than $1000 do not have to be itemized. If animals are to be purchased, state the species and the number to be used.

Travel

Itemize travel requests and justify on Form Page 5. Provide the purpose and destination of each trip and the number of individuals for whom funds are requested.

Patient care costs

If inpatient and/or outpatient costs are requested for research with human subjects, provide the names of any hospitals and/or clinics and the amounts requested for each on Form Page 5.

State whether each hospital or clinic has a currently effective DHHS-negotiated research patient care rate agreement and, if not, what basis is used for calculating costs. If an applicant does not have a DHHS-negotiated rate, the PHS awarding component can approve a provisional rate. Indicate, in detail, the basis for estimating costs in this category, including the number of patient days, estimated cost per day, and cost per test or treatment. If both inpatient and outpatient costs are requested, provide information for each separately. If multiple sites are to be used, provide detailed information by site.

Include information regarding projected patient accrual for the project/budget periods and relate this information to the budget request for patient care costs. If patient accrual is anticipated to be lower at the start or during the course of the project, plan budget(s) accordingly.

Provide specific information regarding anticipated sources of other support for patient care costs, for example, third party recovery or pharmaceutical companies. Include any potential or expected utilization of General Clinical Research Centers/Clinical Translation Science Awards.

Alterations and renovations

Itemize by category and justify on Form Page 5 the costs of essential alterations and renovations including repairs, painting, removal or installation of partitions, shielding, or air conditioning. Where applicable, provide the square footage and costs. Note, costs for any Alterations and Renovations (A&R) were previously unallowable from foreign institutions, international organizations and domestic applications with foreign subawards. However, an HHS policy change now allows for minor A&R (<$500,000) on these applications. When requesting minor A&R costs under this policy, provide detailed information on the planned A&R in the budget justification.

Other expenses

Itemize any other expenses by category and unit cost. These might include animal maintenance (unit care costs and number of care days), patient travel, patient participation incentives, donor fees, publication costs, computer charges, rentals and leases, equipment maintenance, service contracts, and tuition remission when budgeted separately from salary/fringe benefits. **Justify costs on Form Page 5.**

Consortium/Contractual costs

Each participating consortium/contractual organization must submit a separate detailed budget for both the initial budget period (Form Page 4), and the entire proposed project period (Form Page 5).

Consortium arrangements may involve personnel costs, supplies, and other allowable costs, including Facilities and Administrative (F&A) costs. Contractual costs for support services, such as the laboratory testing of biological materials, clinical services, or data processing, are occasionally sufficiently high to warrant a similar categorical breakdown of costs.

For each budget from a participating consortium/contractual organization, leave the "Consortium/Contractual Direct Costs" category blank and use the "Subtotal Direct Costs" category to total the consortium direct costs. When F&A costs are requested by a consortium organization, enter those costs in the "Consortium/Contractual F&A Costs" category for each supplementary budget. Provide the F&A cost base and rate information in the budget justification section. The "Total Direct Costs for Initial Budget Period" category can be used for the consortium/contractual Total Costs (Direct Costs plus F&A).

For the applicant organization budget, list the sum of all consortium/contractual costs (direct and F&A). Insert additional budget page(s) after Form Page 5, numbering them sequentially. (Do not use 5a, 5b, 5c, etc.)

Source Document Visit Note Template

IRB # _____

Title: _____

_____

Principal Investigator: _____

VISIT PROGRESS NOTE

Date: _____ **Visit Number:** _____ **Subject ID #:** _____

Contact with: _____

HEALTH STATUS

Weight: _____

BP: _____ Temperature: _____ Pulse: _____ Respiration: _____

LABS

Blood drawn (initials/date/time): _____

Urine collection (date/time): _____

ADVERSE EVENTS

Symptoms/Complaint   Date Started   Date Ended (or Ongoing)

_____

_____

_____

EMERGENCY ROOM VISIT OR HOSPITALIZATION

Has there been an ER visit or hospitalization since the last visit?

_____ Yes   _____ No

If yes, date(s) and reason: _____

_____

Records requested (initials & date): _____

CONCOMITANT MEDICATIONS

Drug	Dose/Frequency	Date Started	Date Ended	Reason

NOTES:

_____

_____

_____

_____

_____

_____

Research Coordinator   Principal Investigator

_____   _____

Date   Date

Data and Safety Monitoring Plan (DSMP) Template

General instructions

- The DSMP should be a concise summary of the plan for monitoring:
  - The research data,
  - The safety of participants, and
  - The appropriate conduct of clinical research.
- The plan should be written in a manner understandable to physicians, scientists, and nonscientists. Technical language and abbreviations should be defined.
- The section headings provided below should be used.
- The format guidelines for the DSMP are:
  - A 12-point font and
  - Two to three pages in length, although the length may vary.

Study title

Specify the formal study title.

Type of research data or events to be monitored

Describe the type of data or events to be captured under the monitoring plan (e.g., study accruals, protocol deviations, protocol violations, unanticipated problems, adverse events, and changes in risk/benefit).

Methods and frequency of analysis

Describe the plan to be followed by the principal investigator/study staff to ensure the safety of participants, the appropriate conduct of research and the integrity of safety and/or efficacy data. Include the methods and frequency of analysis. Attach a copy of data collection forms (if any).

Person(s) responsible for data monitoring

1. Specify the name(s) and role(s) of the person(s) responsible for monitoring the data collected. Depending on the risk, size, and complexity of the study, the investigator, a group of experts, an independent Data and Safety Monitoring Board (DSMB)/Data and Safety Monitoring Committee (DSMC), and/or others may be assigned primary responsibility for the monitoring activity.
2. Specify the name and role of the person responsible for submitting reports of unanticipated problems, adverse events, protocol deviations, and protocol violations to the

IRB and indicated entities (e.g., NIH, FDA, sponsor). When the investigator is the sponsor of the IND/IDE, include the plan for reporting adverse events to the FDA and, when applicable, to investigators at other sites.

Reporting unanticipated problems, adverse events, protocol deviations, and protocol violations

1. Describe the plan to be followed by the principal investigator/study staff for the review and reporting of: adverse events experienced by participants under their care, untoward events occurring during the course of the study, and (when applicable) sponsor safety reports and/or DSMB reports.
2. Specify the procedure and time frames for reporting to the IRB, study sponsor and/or indicated entities.

Stopping rules

1. Define the specific stopping rules. Stopping rules are predetermined guidelines to determine that the study should be altered or stopped based on review of study-related events (e.g., failure to meet study accrual goals, study endpoints). For example, studies may be stopped when there is greater than expected morbidity and/or mortality rates or when the experimental arm in a comparison study is shown to be better or worse statistically than the standard care arm.
2. Describe the nature of the action(s) indicated by the specific stopping rule.

Procedures and time frames for communicating outcomes   Specify the procedure and time frames for communicating outcomes of monitoring reviews to the IRB, study sponsor, and/or indicated entities.

Precautions for maintaining data integrity   Describe the plan to be followed by the principal investigator/study staff to monitor adherence to the IRB-approved protocol and to assure the validity and integrity of the data.

Page numbers followed by f, t, and b indicate figures, tables, and boxes, respectively.